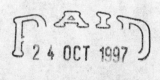

MCQs in Anatomy

A Self-testing Supplement to 'Essential Anatomy'

J. S. P. Lumley MS FRCS FMAA(Hon) FGA

Professor of Vascular Surgery, University of London;
Honorary Consultant Surgeon, St Bartholomew's Hospital,
London; Past Examiner in Anatomy for the Royal College of
Surgeons of England

J. L. Craven BSc MD FRCS

Consultant Surgeon, District General Hospital, York;
Examiner in Pathology for the Royal College of Surgeons
of England

Both formerly Assistant Lecturers at University College

THIRD EDITION

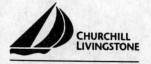

CHURCHILL
LIVINGSTONE

NEW YORK EDINBURGH LONDON MADRID MELBOURNE SAN FRANCISCO TOKYO 1996

CHURCHILL LIVINGSTONE
Medical Division of Pearson Professional Limited

Distributed in the United States of America by
Churchill Livingstone Inc., 650 Avenue of the Americas,
New York, N.Y. 10011, and by associated companies,
branches and representatives throughout the world.

First edition 1979
Second edition 1988
Third edition 1996

Standard Edition ISBN 0443 04977 7

British Library Cataloguing in Publication Data
A catalogue record for this book is available from the British Library

Library of Congress Cataloging in Publication Data
A Catalog record for this book is available from the
Library of Congress

International Student Edition first published 1989
International Student Edition of 3rd edition published 1996

ISBN 0443 056145

Produced by Longman Singapore Publishers Pte Ltd
Printed in Singapore

Contents

Preface to the Third Edition

The production of the third edition of *MCQs in Anatomy* is timed to follow the publication of the fifth edition of *Essential Anatomy*, its companion volume.

The new edition contains additional clinical material and the text has been revised throughout. The embryology chapter has been removed but the embryology of individual organs expanded where appropriate.

The format of the questions has been changed from four to five options. This is in keeping with the style of the majority of current MCQ examinations. It has also provided the opportunity to increase the assessment and the information included in each area covered.

J. S. P. L.
J. L. C.

Introduction

Objective testing

The perfect examination would be one in which the student was accurately assessed in his knowledge, comprehension, application, analysis and evaluation of material pertinent to the subject being examined. The use of the essay type question paper as the sole means of assessment has been criticised because of its reliance on subjective qualities.

For several years educationalists of many different disciplines have sought methods of objective testing which examined all the above mentioned qualities. In all objective tests the student has to choose the correct response out of one or more alternatives, his answers being either right or wrong. The subjective judgement of the examiner thus plays no part in this form of examination. Objective testing has been used extensively in the U.S.A. since the end of the Second World War, but introduction in the U.K. has been slow, and it has reached the universities generally via schools and technical colleges. However, multiple choice question papers are now in use in most medical schools and it has been necessary for both the medical student and his teacher to become fully acquainted with the uses and abuses of this testing technique. It is appropriate here to consider the merits of the various examination techniques and, perhaps most important, to compare objective testing with the traditional essay question.

The essay

Students and examiners have questioned the effectiveness of an essay paper in measuring the attainment of a number of years of study. The area covered by such an examination is very limited, the more so when a wide choice of questions is allowed. It thus encourages the students to 'spot questions' and to concentrate on only part of the syllabus. The marking of essays is time consuming and unreliable, there being variations in an individual examiner's reassessment of papers as well as between examiners. This variation makes comparison on a national level difficult and is further accentuated by what has been described as the deep psychological reluctance of examiners to allocate more than seventy per cent of the total marks allowed for any given essay question. However, the essay does determine the candidate's ability to write clear and legible English, it tests his ability to collect and quantitate material, and it assesses his powers of logic, original thought and creativity. In terms of cost the essay question is cheap to produce but it is expensive to mark.

The composition of objective questions

The objective form of examination is best composed by a panel of examiners, each having a complete understanding of the syllabus and a thorough knowledge of the field of study. The panel must first decide the parts of the syllabus to be covered by the examination, and the level of knowledge required by the candidate. The type of objective test and the number of options per question is decided and each member of the panel prepares a set of questions for the group to consider. A multiple choice question consists of a stem (the initial question) and four or more options; one of these options in the multiple choice question is correct and this is known as the key, the incorrect responses being known as the distractors. In the case of multiple response questions, there may be more than one correct response. (This form of question has also been termed multiple completion, multiple answer, multiple true or false and the indeterminate response by various authorities, but in most centres, and in this text, it will subsequently be referred to as a multiple choice question.)

Stem and options should be brief, using the minimum number of words, and the instructions should be clear and simple, the language used being appropriate to the verbal ability and requirement of the candidate. The question must be of some educational value. The words 'always' and 'never' should be avoided and the stem should preferably not be in the negative. There should be no recurrent phrase in the options which can be included in the stem. The key (the correct option or options) must be wholly correct and unambiguous. It is important for the correct response to be in different positions in each of a group of questions and some form of random allocation may be necessary. The distractors (the wrong options) are the most exacting and challenging part of objective question composition and the standard of an objective test is probably best assessed in terms of the quality of its distractors. They must always be plausible, yet completely wrong. They should be in a parallel style to the key and they should not contain clues. Common misconceptions form good distractors. 'None of them' or 'all of them' are not satisfactory distractors. Four options are thought by many authorities to be sufficient.

After the draft questions have been collected, it is advisable for a panel of examiners to assess their value and limitations. Inaccurate and irrelevant material is then excluded. Even the most experienced of examiners will find that a panel will offer constructive criticism on the majority of his questions. Ideally, once the panel has accepted a series of questions these should be pre-tested on a group of students and the results analysed. It is desirable for a question to have been pre-tested on 300 to 400 students before it comes into regular use in a qualifying examination. The difficulty of a question can be determined by calculating the percentage of students giving the right answer, and its discriminatory value (the ratio of correct/incorrect responses) calculated in a manner which takes into account whether or not the better students obtained the correct response. The facility value (difficulty index) records the percentage of correct responses and compares it with the total number of candidates. Additional information on the mean and range of distribution of the answers can also be obtained with a discriminatory index and a bi-serial correlation coefficient (relating the total candidate response to an option, with the results of the top 27 per cent and the bottom 27 per cent of the candidates to the same option). Figures for both the discriminatory index and the bi-serial correlation coefficient range from plus 1 to minus 1. Questions with factors of less than 0.20 should be rejected (unless a few difficult or easy questions are to be included). Values of 0.21 to 0.29 are of marginal discriminatory value. The values 0.30 to 0.39 show a reasonable discriminatory power of the option, whereas results greater than 0.44 indicate good discrimination by a question of the candidates under test. The effectiveness of the question is also measured in terms of the number of students attempting it — the value of a question certainly cannot be assessed if a large number of students leave it out. Computer printouts on a series of questions will also provide the ranking of students, the scatter of the results and a raw score (i.e. the number of correct, less the number of incorrect results).

The pre-testing, though very time consuming, greatly adds to the validity and reliability of the objective test. Using the results of these tests the panel can rephrase unsatisfactory questions and compile the definitive examination paper. The time allowed in the pre-test is not limited but the students are asked to note the time taken to complete the test; the time required for the final version is thus arrived at. This time should allow at least 90 per cent of the candidates to complete the paper. It is usual to start an examination paper with a few easier questions (i.e. with a low difficulty index) and similarly a few difficult questions can be included at the end. It has been found that a good (wide) range of results is obtained by setting a large number of questions with average discrimination rather than including a large number with high or low discriminatory indices. Testing of the questions should not stop after the pre-testing phase, the information gained from each subsequent examination should be used to review continuously all the question material.

Obviously a series of questions which have been pre-tested and shown to be satisfactory is of great value to the examiner. Such questions can be used repeatedly provided they have not been freely available to the students. Security is an important factor, particularly when the number of questions is small and does not cover the whole syllabus. For this reason it is advisable to have a large number of questions available. It is reasonable to assume that if a student is capable of memorising the correct responses to a large number of questions (even if these are known to him) he will also have a passable knowledge of the syllabus.

A satisfactory bank of questions takes three to five years to build. After this time the questions can be grouped into sections and, whenever an examination paper is required, questions can be chosen at random from each section. Continuous updating and revision of this material should be undertaken and new material added regularly. The history of each question in the bank should be recorded. Repetitive use of the questions over a number of years allows annual standards to be compared.

The student's approach to objective testing

Any student required to undertake an objective test for a qualifying examination or a postgraduate examination should ensure he has some preliminary experience in this form of testing. It is essential for him to know and have sampled the style of questions used by his particular examining board.

In any objective test all the instructions provided must be carefully read and understood and the student's designated number marked in the appropriate section, otherwise a computer marking system will reject the paper — this will not impress the examining authority.

The type of objective test used in medical education does vary and some of these types have already been discussed. Whatever form the question takes in the objective test, it is essential that the student starts on his first quick 'run' through the questions by filling in all the answers he knows to be correct. On this first 'run' he should also mark (on the paper) the questions where he is fully acquainted with the material but is unsure of the correct response. On the second 'run' all his attention can now be given to this group of questions, in which he should be able to make an informed guess. Experience has shown that his chances of being correct in this situation are above average. He should, as one examiner expresses it, 'play his hunches'. The questions which he does not understand are probably best left unanswered as at best he can only hope for a 50 per cent chance of a correct response on a random basis in the true/false situation, and only a 25 per cent chance of a correct response in a four item multiple choice question. In multiple choice questions the marking is usually positive, a mark being given for a correct answer and none for an incorrect one. In multiple response questions (as in this text) a mark is given for each correct response, whether this be true or false, and usually a mark is subtracted for each incorrect response. Most examination systems have now abolished the use of a correction factor for guessing as this was found to have little effect on the ranking of the candidates, and it has also been realised that informed guessing is in itself a useful discrimination.

Lack of time is not usually a problem in medical objective testing. Since these tests are of the 'power' rather than the 'speed' variety, i.e. knowledge rather than ability against the clock is being tested. Excessive time may be a disadvantage to the candidate as repeated reassessment of the answers may distract from the correct response rather than produce improvement. In the multiple choice situation it has been found that one minute is usually necessary per question although more time is required to answer a question containing a number of distractors.

Transcribing 300 items from a question paper to an answer sheet (i.e. 60 questions each with 5 options) takes a minimum of 10 minutes and the habit of leaving such transcriptions to the end of an examination is best avoided since, if rushed, it may introduce unnecessary inaccuracies.

Etymological hazards
The rarity of absolutes in anatomy means that a large variety of adjectives and adverbs are commonly used in its description. These increase the difficulty of both setting and answering multiple choice questions. Although one can question the desirability of assessing knowledge which is dependent on the 'strength of an adjective', these adjectives do form the language of present day medical practice. This factor is borne out by their use in some questions and answers of the present text. Nevertheless, the

examiner must avoid ambiguity and in addition his questions must not contain clues to the correct answer. Such terms as 'invariable', 'always', 'must', 'all', 'only', and 'never' should be avoided since they imply absolutes and are therefore likely to be wrong.

The terms 'may' and 'can' also give rise to ambiguity. In anatomy almost anything 'may occur' and statements using this phrase are unlikely to be completely wrong. If these terms are used and the student is able to answer that the question 'certainly may' or 'certainly may not', he has little chance of being wrong. The term 'sometimes' comes into the same category.

The adjectives and adverbs 'common', 'usual', 'frequent' (commonly, usually, frequently), 'likely' and 'often' are an integral part of everyday medical language but their use in the multiple choice question may also lead to ambiguity. Their meanings are very similar yet their values depend largely on the context of the question. Expressed as incidences they may well range from 30 to 70 per cent. They may be considerably modified by the addition of 'quite', 'most', 'very' and 'extremely'. The examiner must be particularly careful of his choice of these terms. The 'majority' implies more than 50 per cent, whereas the 'vast majority' implies nearly 100 per cent.

The term 'typical' is a useful one for multiple choice questions. Its meaning implies 'that which is found most commonly'. 'Characteristic' implies a time honoured anatomical feature, and 'recognised' an accepted textbook description. Further vague terminology used in medical practice yet best avoided in the multiple choice question includes 'associated with', 'accompanied by', 'related to', 'linked with' and 'lend support to'.

On the negative side, 'uncommon', 'unusual', 'infrequent' (uncommonly, unusually, infrequently), 'unlikely' and 'rare' are all terms commonly used yet their use in the multiple choice question must not give rise to ambiguity. As with their positive equivalents they are markedly influenced by the addition of such terms as 'most' and 'very'. The term 'significant' is best kept for its statistical use and the terms 'increased' and 'more' should be restricted to direct comparative situations.

In conclusion, words used in multiple choice questions, although giving rise to apparent ambiguity, remain those in common use in medical practice; both the examiner and the student must be fully conversant with their meanings and disadvantages in order to avoid any confusion. It is hoped that the questions which follow will also help in this regard.

How to use this book

The text, consisting of questions and answers ('true or false'), is arranged throughout in such a way that all questions appear on left-hand pages and all answers on right-hand pages.

In use the student may conveniently cover the right-hand page with a blank sheet on which to note down the answers for comparison.

I   The Structure of the Body

1   **The cell membrane:**
  a   is approximately 7 nm thickness.   (   )
  b   is capable of selective permeability.   (   )
  c   allows passage of specific ions through
       carbohydrate-gated channels.   (   )
  d   is activated by a secondary messenger system.   (   )

  e   may discharge particles by a process of vacuolation. (   ) .

2   **Covered cytoplasmic inclusions:**
  a   contain cytosol.   (   )

  b   together comprise the cell cytoskeleton.   (   )

  c   are concerned with the carbohydrate metabolism.   (   )

  d   are concerned with the collection and transport of
       cellular elements and chemicals.   (   )
  e   are involved in phagocytosis.   (   )

3   **The cell nucleus:**
  a   is usually 4 to 10 μm across.   (   )

  b   is the site of RNA synthesis.   (   )
  c   is surrounded by a single layered membrane.   (   )

  d   contains nucleoli responsible for the production
       of the mitotic spindles during cell division.   (   )
  e   contains ribosomes.   (   )

4   **Cells are united by:**
  a   desmosomes.   (   )
  b   intermediate junction.   (   )
  c   tight junctions.   (   )
  d   gated junctions.   (   )
  e   terminal junctions.   (   )

a T— The membrane is protein-lined double lipid layer.
b T— It actively regulates the internal cellular environment.
c F— The channels are protein-gated.

d F— Stimulation of the surface of the cell membrane activates
      the secondary messenger system, these mediators acting
      within the cell.
e T— The process of endocytosis.

a F— This is the cytoplasm outside the membrane covered
      inclusions.
b F— This is a heterogenous collection of filamentous structures
      within the cytosol.
c T— The endoplasmic reticulum carrying out this function also
      subserves lipid metabolism and detoxification.
d T— The Golgi apparatus subserves these functions.

e T— The mitochondria subserve this function.

a T— The cells vary from 5 to 50 μm, the limited size facilitates
      the rapid diffusion of metabolites through their structure.
b T— The nuclear DNA serves as a template for this process.
c F— The nuclear membrane has two layers, the outer being
      part of the endoplasmic reticulum.
d F— Nucleoli contain specific chromosome fragments
      responsible for replication of RNA.
e T— These can cross the nuclear membrane to sites of protein
      synthesis.

a T— Desmosomes are small button-like areas on the cell
b T   membrane, they provide the strongest form of anchorage.
c T   In intermediate junctions, the gap is retained but a cobweb
d F   of filaments extends into the cytoplasm of the adjacent
e F   cells. In tight junctions, the intercellular gap is lost; these
       are areas of great cellular permeability.

5   Epithelial tissue:
a gives rise to the sebaceous glands of the scalp.   (   )
b undergoes constant renewal in most regions of the
   alimentary tract.   (   )
c lining the urinary tract contains numerous goblet
   cells.   (   )
d lining the respiratory tract is keratinised.   (   )

e can be resistant to harmful metabolites.   (   )

6   Exocrine glands:
a typically discharge their contents directly into
   the blood stream.   (   )
b usually secretes in a holocrine manner.   (   )

c are of mesenchymal origin.   (   )
d are absent in stratified squamous epithelium.   (   )

e may be unicellular.   (   )

7   Elastic fibres are:
a prominent in hyaline cartilage.   (   )

b formed from fibroblasts.   (   )

c prominent in superficial fascia.   (   )
d prominent in aponeuroses.   (   )
e prominent in retinacula.   (   )

8   Hyaline cartilage:
a contains a few fine collagen-like fibres.   (   )
b is the bony precursor in cartilaginous ossification.   (   )

c unites the sphenoid and occipital bones in the child.   (   )

d forms the knee menisci.   (   )
e is particularly vascular in relation to joints.   (   )

a T— And to most other glands.

b T— The alimentary tract is lined by simple epithelium between the oesophagus and the anal canal.

c F— The transitional epithelium of the urinary contains few glands.

d F— The lining is mostly ciliated columnar epithelium with numerous goblet cells.

e T— It can serve as a selective barrier and can also be resistant to chemicals.

a F— This is the definition of an endocrine gland. Exocrine glands have ducts opening on to a surface.

b F— Most exocrine glands secrete without damage to the cell, i.e. merocrine or epicrine secretion, as do most endocrine glands.

c F— They are of epithelial origin.

d F— Sebaceous and sweat glands are common in this form of tissue.

e T— Goblet cells are unicellular.

a F— Hyaline cartilage contains many cells and a few fine collagen-like fibres in the matrix.

b T— And found mainly in some ligaments attached to vertebrae.

c F— This tissue is a mixture of fat and collagen fibres.

d F— These are formed mainly of collagen fibres.

e F— These are thickenings of the deep fascia related to joints and are formed mainly of collagen fibres.

a T— And is found in synovial joints and in costal cartilages.

b T— Ossification in mesenchyme takes place on a fibrous tissue model.

c T— Growth in length of the skull occurs mainly at this joint; bony fusion occurring after the appearance of the last molar tooth, about the 25th year.

d F— These are formed of fibrocartilage.

e F— It is an avascular firm tissue of chondrocytes in an abundant matrix.

9 Long bones:
a usually ossify in mesenchyme. ( )
b consist entirely of compact bone. ( )

c normally contain yellow marrow. ( )
d are organised in Haversian systems. ( )

e are covered with the acellular periosteum. ( )

10 Cartilaginous ossification:
a occurs in all long bones except the clavicle. ( )

b occurs in cartilage which has replaced a
membranous model. ( )
c has its primary centres appearing at about the
18th week of intra-uterine life. ( )
d secondary centres typically fuse at puberty. ( )

e is typical in the bones of the skull vault. ( )

11 In the development of a long bone:
a osteoblasts come to line the primary alveoli. ( )
b osteoblasts become the osteocytes. ( )
c ossification extends along the body of the bone
as endochondral ossification. ( )
d the epiphyseal plate separates the metaphysis
from the diaphysis. ( )
e circumferential growth is from the diaphyseal
centre. ( )

12 The epiphyses:
a are all present at birth. ( )
b are formed in hyaline cartilage. ( )

c are present in all long bones. ( )
d contribute to growth in length and girth of long
bones. ( )
e may occur at sites of muscle attachment. ( )

a F— Long bones usually ossify in hyaline cartilage.
b F— Compact bone is found in the body of the bone but cancellous bone occupies most of the ends of the bones.
c T— In the healthy adult the marrow is of the yellow variety.
d T— Bone is laid down in concentric layers centripetally. Small blood vessels are usually found in the middle.
e F— The thick fibrous periosteum contains many granular, bone forming, osteoblasts.

a T— The clavicle has a mixed mesenchymal and cartilaginous ossification.
b T— The cartilage is of the hyaline type.
c F— These usually appear in the 8th week of intrauterine life.
d F— Secondary centres usually appear between birth and puberty, and fuse about the 18th–20th year.
e F— These undergo mesenchymal ossification, usually starting at the 5th and 6th weeks of intrauterine life.

a F— Osteoblasts line the larger secondary alveoli formed by the
b T   osteoclasts absorbing the calcified matrix of the cartilage.
c T— The cartilage model is gradually replaced by bone.
d F— The epiphyseal plate lies between the epiphysis and the metaphysis.
e F— This is by subperiosteal ossification.

a F— These are secondary centres of ossification and formed by
b T   osteoblasts: only those of the knee are present at birth. Most of the remainder appear by puberty.
c T
d F— The increase in girth of a long bone occurs by the laying down of bone by the periosteum.
e T— Pressure and atavistic epiphyses also exist.

13 **Primary cartilaginous joints:**
a unite the lower end of the tibia and fibula. ( )
b occur between the teeth and jaw. ( )

c comprise the sutures of the vault of the skull. ( )
d unite the two pubic bones. ( )

e include the costochondral junctions. ( )

14 **In synovial joints the:**
a articular surfaces are all lined by hyaline cartilage. ( )

b fibrocartilaginous discs usually partially divide the
joint cavity. ( )
c hinged variety is exemplified by the
metacarpophalangeal joints. ( )

d stability of the joint is generally inversely related to
its mobility. ( )
e hip joint is of the saddle variety. ( )

15 **Striated (voluntary) muscle:**
a contains alternating A and Z bands. ( )

b fibres are multinucleate. ( )
c is present in the upper part of the oesophagus. ( )

d fibres are bound together by the sarcolemma. ( )

e is predominantly supplied from lateral horn
efferent fibres. ( )

a **F**— Primary cartilaginous joints are found between the body
b **F**   of a long bone and its epiphyses. The unions in a, b, and c
c **F**   are all examples of fibrous joints.
d **F**— The pubic bones are united by a secondary cartilaginous
       joint (symphysis).
e **T**

a **F**— The temporomandibular and sternoclavicular joints are
       exceptions and are both lined by fibrocartilage. Their discs
       completely divide the joint into two cavities.
b **F**— But see (a).

c **F**— These are ellipsoid joints capable of abduction, adduction
       and circumduction as well as flexion and extension. The
       interphalangeal joints are true hinge joints.
d **T**— The shoulder joint is the most mobile but most easily
       dislocated.
e **F**— This is ball and socket joint; the carpometacarpal joint of
       the thumb is a saddle joint.

a **F**— The muscle is formed of alternating A and I bands, the Z
       disc dividing the latter.
b **T**— The nuclei are peripherally arranged.
c **T**— Also in the anal canal. The remainder of the alimentary
       tract has smooth muscle in its wall.
d **F**— Fibres are surrounded by the sarcolemma and attached to
       their neighbours by the fibrous endomysium. Bundles are
       enclosed in the perimysium.
e **F**— The motor nerve supplying it is from the anterior horn
       cells of the spinal cord and brain stem.

16 **In muscular activity:**
 a a synergistic muscle is one that relaxes against the pull of gravity. ( )

 b a parallel arrangement of fibres provides a more powerful movement than an oblique arrangement. ( )

 c antagonistic muscles oppose the prime movers. ( )
 d innervation is by the muscle spindles. ( )

 e Impulses from sensory endings pass into the posterior horn of the spinal cord. ( )

17 **A nerve fibre:**
 a in the central nervous system has astrocytes forming the axon sheath. ( )
 b consists of an axon, usually covered with a myelin sheath. ( )
 c ends as 'boutons'. ( )

 d in a peripheral nerve may be injured and then recover. ( )

 e in the central nervous system is devoid of cellular inclusions. ( )

18 **Neuroglia:**
 a exist only in the brain. ( )
 b are cellular neural connective tissue. ( )

 c have a phagocytic function. ( )
 d produce myelin. ( )

 e are concerned with the nutrition of neurons. ( )

19 **The spinal nerves:**
 a are formed from dorsal and ventral roots, each root with both sensory and motor fibres. ( )
 b are distributed to the limbs partly through their dorsal rami. ( )

 c leave the vertebral canal via the intervertebral foramina. ( )
 d have ganglia on the ventral roots. ( )

 e comprise 31 pairs. ( )

a F— During muscular activity prime movers produce movement at joints while synergists steady other joints. Relaxation against gravity is known as paradoxical movement.
b F— In muscles of equal volume a parallel arrangement gives greater range of movement but less power than an oblique arrangement.
c T— And control the rate and range of movement.
d F— Primary innervation of a muscle fibre is by the motor end plate; muscle spindles are sensory stretch receptors.
e T

a F— Oligodendroglia cells have this function which Schwann cells perform in the peripheral nervous system.
b T— There are also many unmyelinated fibres.
c T— These are related to the processes and cell bodies of adjacent nerves, the union being called a synapse.
d T— Schwann cells play an important role in this regeneration. Little or no regeneration occurs in the central nervous system.
e F— Neurons possess large nuclei and prominent cellular inclusions.

a T— Neuroglia do not exist outside the brain and comprise
b T three different types of cells: astrocytes, oligodendroglia and microglia.
c T— The microglia are small mobile phagocytes and
d T oligodendroglia produce the myelin of the central nervous system.
e T

a F— The dorsal roots contain sensory and the ventral, motor fibres.
b F— The limbs receive their nerve supply from the brachial and lumbosacral plexuses, these being formed from ventral rami.
c T— The foramina are formed by adjacent vertebrae. The first cervical nerve passes laterally above the first vertebra.
d F— The ganglia are the neurons of sensory fibres and are found on the dorsal roots.
e T— 8 cervical, 12 thoracic, 5 lumbar, 5 sacral and 1 coccygeal.

20   The autonomic nervous system:

a   supplies the glands, smooth muscle and cardiac muscle.   (   )

b   rises from the special visceral column of the spinal cord.   (   )

c   has peripheral ganglia near the walls of the organ it supplies.   (   )

d   prepares the body for fight and flight.   (   )

e   has no distribution to the lower limbs.   (   )

21   The sympathetic nervous system:

a   has myelinated postganglionic fibres passing from the sympathetic trunk to the spinal nerves.   (   )

b   has trunks extending from the base of the skull to the coccyx.   (   )

c   has usually only five ganglia in the sympathetic trunk.   (   )

d   fibres passing to the head and neck leave the spinal cord in the 5th–8th cervical spinal nerves.   (   )

e   sends preganglionic fibres to the cortex of the suprarenal gland.   (   )

22   The parasympathetic nervous system:

a   receives its fibres from nuclei associated with the 3rd, 5th, 7th and 10th cranial nerves.   (   )

b   receives its pelvic outflow from the 2nd, 3rd and 4th lumbar segments.   (   )

c   has its peripheral ganglia usually in the walls of the organ being supplied.   (   )

d   sends an innervation to the suprarenal medulla.   (   )

e   carries no afferent fibres.   (   )

a T— It is not under voluntary control.

b F— It arises from the general visceral column. The special
visceral column of the brain stem supplies striated
(voluntary) muscle derived from the pharyngeal arches.

c T— Parasympathetic ganglia are situated in this position,
sympathetic ganglia lie in the sympathetic trunk, usually
away from the organ.

d T— This is a general description of sympathetic activity.
Parasympathetic governs more vegetative functions. It is
responsible for evacuation of gut and urinary bladder and
slows the heart rate.

e F— Peripheral smooth muscle (e.g. in the arterial walls and
glands such as sweat glands) receives autonomic
innervation.

a F— The preganglionic fibres are myelinated, the postganglionic
are unmyelinated, these respectively representing the
white and grey rami communicantes.

b T

c F— The trunk usually has 3 cervical, 10 thoracic, 4 lumbar, and
4 sacral ganglia.

d F— Fibres passing to the head and neck come mainly from the
first thoracic segment, synapse in the cervical ganglia and
are distributed mostly with the branches of the carotid
arteries, and the spinal and cardiac nerves.

e T— The medulla of the gland does receive a dense innervation
of these fibres.

a F— Although the 5th nerve distributes parasympathetic fibres
derived from the 7th and 9th cranial nerves it is alone in
having none at its origin. The others have.

b F— Pelvic outflow comes from 2nd, 3rd and 4th sacral
segments of the spinal cord.

c T— The exceptions are the cranial parasympathetic ganglia
which are separated from their organs.

d F— The suprarenal medulla receives preganglionic sympathetic
fibres.

e F— Afferent (e.g. pain fibres from the viscera) pathways are
present in both sympathetic and parasympathetic systems.

23   The white blood cells:
a   have coarse granules when of the basophil variety. ( )
b   have pale basophilic cytoplasm in the
lymphocyte variety. ( )
c   have lobulated nuclei in the neutrophils. ( )
d   are most commonly of the neutrophil variety. ( )
e   pass out of the blood stream and take part in
the inflammatory response. ( )

24   Red bone marrow:
a   is present in most bones at birth. ( )
b   exists in the adult only in the long bones. ( )

c   contains precursors of both erythrocytes and
white blood cells. ( )
d   contains precursors of blood platelets. ( )
e   is composed of a coarse fibrous network. ( )

25   Reduction of the blood supply to an area:
a   is known as ischaemia. ( )
b   is a feature of the inflammatory response. ( )
c   may lead to infarction. ( )

d   is commonly the result of thrombosis. ( )
e   may be the result of an embolus. ( )

26   The lymph nodes:
a   receive afferent lymph vessels at the hilus. ( )
b   have a fine reticular network of collagen fibres. ( )
c   have a peripheral subcapsular space. ( )
d   have an inner densely packed medulla. ( )

e   are surrounded by an elastic capsule. ( )

a T— White cells are nucleated and either granular (e.g.
b T   neutrophils) or agranular (e.g. lymphocytes).

c T
d T
e T— Being involved in the classical features of swelling, pain, redness and heat.

a T— Red bone marrow is present in most bones at birth, but
b T   fatty yellow marrow gradually replaces it in the shafts of long bones so that, in the adult, red marrow remains mainly in the vertebrae, ribs, sternum and flat bones.
c T— It contains precursors of all the cellular and noncellular elements of the blood.
d T
e F— It is composed of a reticular network of fine collagen fibres.

a T
b F— In this response blood flow is increased.
c T— This term indicates death of an area of tissue which may then become infected and putrified, a condition known as gangrene.
d T— Blood clotting on the wall of a vessel and occluding the
e T— lumen is called a thrombus. When the clot moves, it is called an embolus.

a F— Afferent vessels enter the convexity of the node and
b T   efferent vessels leave the hilus on the concave side.
c T— Into which the afferent vessels open.
d F— The outer cortex is densely packed with cells and follicles, the central medulla is loosely packed with cells.
e F— The capsule is fibrous and from it, fibrous trabeculae pass inwards.

II The Vertebral Column

27 **In the vertebral column:**
   a the individual vertebrae are all separately
      identifiable in the adult.   (   )
   b cervical vertebrae all have bifid spines.   (   )

   c thoracic vertebrae all have articular surfaces
      for ribs.   (   )

   d the articular processes arise near the junction
      of the vertebral body and its pedicles.   (   )
   e primary fetal curvatures are retained in the
      thoracic and sacral regions.   (   )

28 **In the cervical region:**
   a the atlas vertebra has no body.   (   )

   b the superior articular facets of the axis face
      anterolaterally.   (   )
   c the 6th cervical spine is the most prominent.   (   )
   d dislocation of the dens is prevented by the alar
      and apical ligaments.   (   )

   e the upper vertebrae lie behind the oropharynx.   (   )

29 **The intervertebral discs:**
   a are largely composed of hyaline cartilage.   (   )
   b the anulus fibrosus is formed of elastic tissue.   (   )

   c contribute about one quarter of the length of
      the vertebral column.   (   )

   d are found in all regions of the vertebral column.   (   )

   e may compress the spinal cord when injured.   (   )

a **F**— Five vertebrae fuse together and form the sacrum, and others form the coccyx.

b **F**— All have a foramen in the transverse process. C1 has no spine and C7 is not usually bifid.

c **T**— Lumbar vertebrae are identified by having neither a foramen in the transverse process nor articular facets for ribs.

d **F**— They arise near the junction of the pedicles and the laminae.

e **T**— Secondary curvatures develop after birth in the cervical and lumbar regions. These are the most mobile regions and the most liable to injury.

a **T**— This part becomes attached in early fetal life to the axis as the dens.

b **F**— The facets face upwards.

c **F**— C7 is called the vertebrae prominens.

d **F**— The main factor stabilising the joint is the cruciate ligament. If dislocation occurs, the spinal cord may be crushed.

e **T**— Radiographs of the atlanto-occipital and atlanto-axial joints are taken through the open mouth.

a **F**— The discs are fibrocartilage; the centre part is semi-solid,
b **F** the nucleus pulposus, and the outer part, the anulus fibrosus, the latter is formed of fibrous tissue.

c **T**— During the day the discs are compressed. During sleep, water is re-absorbed and the discs restored to their original size.

d **F**— There are no discs in the sacral or coccygeal regions, nor is there one between C1 and C2.

e **T**— Large posterior central herniations may produce this complication. If the herniation occurs at the posterolateral angle, a spinal nerve may be compressed as it lies in the intervertebral foramen.

30 The vertebral bodies are united by:
a anterior and posterior longitudinal ligaments. ( )
b intervertebral discs. ( )

c ligamenta flava. ( )
d intertransverse ligaments. ( )
e interspinous ligaments. ( )

31 In the vertebral canal the:
a dural covering of the spinal cord fuses with the periosteum of adjacent vertebrae. ( )

b spinal cord of an adult ends about the level of the 2nd lumbar vertebra. ( )

c internal vertebral veins have large branches draining the bodies of the vertebrae. ( )

d spinal nerve roots can be followed into their intervertebral foramina where the roots fuse. ( )

e spinal cord cannot be damaged if a needle is inserted between the 1st and 2nd lumbar spines. ( )

III Thorax

32 The thoracic wall:
a has a cartilaginous skeleton. ( )
b is cylindrical in shape. ( )
c is bounded below by the 7th–10th costal cartilages and the 11th and 12th ribs. ( )
d receives its cutaneous nerves via the brachial plexus. ( )

e gives attachment to abdominal wall muscles. ( )

a T— The anterior ligament is a flat band attached to each
b T   vertebral body and disc. The posterior runs from the axis
        to the sacrum and is also attached to each intervertebral
        disc which itself unites the cartilaginous articular surfaces
        of adjacent bodies.
c F— The ligamenta flava, intertransverse and interspinous
d F   ligaments are accessory ligaments and unite the adjacent
e F   laminae, transverse processes and spines respectively.
        They have no attachment to the vertebral bodies.

a F— Between the bony-ligamentous wall of the canal and the
        dura is the fat-filled extradural space with the emerging
        spinal nerves and the internal vertebral venous plexus.
b T— In a child it ends at a lower level.

c T— The marrow of the vertebral bodies is one of the chief
        blood-forming sites throughout life.
d T— In the lower part of the canal, the nerves run with
        increasing obliquity before emerging through the
        intervertebral or sacral foramina. The dorsal root ganglion
        is situated near the point of fusion.
e F— The spinal cord is still present at this level; for a lumbar
        puncture the needle is inserted above or below the spine
        of the 4th lumbar vertebra.

a F— It has a bony-cartilaginous skeleton.
b F— It is 'conical' in shape, narrower superiorly.
c T— These form the costal margin.

d F— It is segmentally innervated via the ventral and dorsal rami
        of the 1st–11th thoracic nerves.
e T— Rectus abdominis, the external and internal oblique, and
        transversus abdominis muscles each gain attachment to
        the anterior or anterolateral part of the costal margin.
        These muscles play an important role in forced respiration.

33   A typical rib:
a   articulates with the vertebral bodies in two places.   (   )
b   is attached to an intervertebral disc.   (   )

c   bears three facets for articulation with the
vertebral column.   (.)

d   has a costal cartilage which articulates with the
sternum by a synovial joint.   (   )

e   is grooved superiorly by the costal groove.   (   )

34   Intercostal arteries:
a   supply only the posterior part of the intercostal
space.   (   )

b   arise from branches of the subclavian artery and
the descending aorta.   (   )
c   arise from branches of the ascending aorta.   (   )
d   supply the spinal cord.   (   )
e   lie inferior to the accompanying nerve in the
intercostal space.   (   )

35   A typical intercostal nerve:
a   is a ventral ramus of a thoracic spinal nerve.   (   )
b   lies in the majority of its course deep to the
internal intercostal muscle.   (   )
c   lies in the majority of its course in the subcostal
groove.   (   )
d   supplies cutaneous branches to the skin of the back.   (   )

e   may supply abdominal wall skin.   (   )

a **T**— Each typical rib bears two facets on its head for articulation
b **T**   with its own vertebra and the one above. The intervening
crest is attached by an intra-articular ligament to the
intervertebral disc.
c **T**— Two facets for the vertebral bodies described above and
one for articulation with the transverse process at the
costotransverse joint.
d **T**— That between the first rib (not a typical rib) and the
sternum is a primary cartilaginous joint, but the joints
between the 2nd and 7th costal cartilages and the sternum
have a synovial cavity.
e **F**— The costal groove, in which lie the intercostal vessels and
nerve, lies inferiorly on the internal surface of the ribs.

a **F**— Each space is supplied by a posterior artery and paired
anterior arteries. The lower two spaces have only posterior
arteries.
b **T**— The first two posterior arteries and all the anterior arteries
arise from branches of the subclavian; the remainder arise
c **T**   from the aorta.
d **T**— Spinal branches arise from the posterior arteries.
e **F**— The nerve lies inferior to its accompanying artery.

a **T**— It has cutaneous and muscular branches.
b **T**— Where the innermost intercostal is deficient, it lies against
the pleura.
c **T**— The artery and the vein separate it from the bone.

d **F**— The skin of the back is supplied by branches of the dorsal
rami.
e **T**— The skin of the anterior abdominal wall is supplied by the
7th to the 12th intercostal nerves.

36   The diaphragm:
a   is attached to the sternum, costal cartilages, the psoas fascia the transversalis fascia, and the vertebral bodies.   (   )

b   is supplied by both the phrenic and intercostal nerves.   (   )
c   increases the horizontal diameter of the chest on contraction.   (   )
d   has an opening in the central tendon for the inferior vena cava.   (   )
e   contracts during micturition.   (   )

37   The diaphragm is pierced by the:
a   splanchnic nerves.   (   )
b   sympathetic trunks.   (   )

c   left phrenic nerve.   (   )

d   gastric nerves.   (   )

e   the lowest intercostal nerves.   (   )

38   During deep respiration:
a   inspiration is aided by the upper ribs being elevated by the scalene muscles.   (   )

b   inspiration is aided by approximation of the upper ribs.   (   )

c   expiration is due to the elastic recoil of lung tissue and the costal cartilages.   (   )

d   expiration is aided by relaxation of the abdominal wall muscles.   (   )
e   there is often fixing of the shoulder girdles.   (   )

22

a **T**— Via the back of the xiphoid, the lowest six costal cartilages, the lateral and medial arcuate ligaments over quadratus abdominis and psoas respectively, and the right and left crura to the upper three (right) and two (left) lumbar vertebrae respectively.

b **T**— Only the phrenic is motor, the intercostal nerves supply sensory branches to the periphery.

c **F**— Contraction results in flattening of the diaphragm and an increase in the vertical diameter of the chest.

d **T**— This opening is to the right of the midline and also transmits the right phrenic nerve.

e **T**— Expulsive acts, such as micturition and defaecation, follow a rise in intra-abdominal pressure produced by simultaneous diaphragmatic and abdominal wall contraction.

a **T**— The splanchnic nerves pierce the crura.

b **F**— The sympathetic trunks pass behind the medial arcuate ligaments.

c **T**— The left phrenic nerve pierces the left dome of the diaphragm.

d **T**— The anterior and posterior gastric nerves are transmitted with the oesophagus through an opening in the muscular part to the left of the midline. Muscle fibres from the right crus of the diaphragm surround the opening.

e **F**— These lie superficial to the diaphragmatic attachments. The subcostal nerve passes behind the lateral cruciate ligament.

a **F**— In deep inspiration, the uppermost ribs are fixed by the scalene muscles. The scalene muscles only elevate the upper ribs in forced inspiration against an obstruction.

b **T**— Fixation of the upper ribs by the scalene muscles allows the intercostal muscles to raise the remaining ribs by movement at their costotransverse joints.

c **T**— The elastic recoil is a major factor in expiration, and this is helped especially in forced respiration by simultaneous contraction of the abdominal wall muscles which also fix the lower ribs.

d **F**— The abdominal muscles contract and push the liver and the diaphragm upwards.

e **T**— This allows serratus anterior and the pectoralis muscles to raise the ribs.

39 The adult female mammary gland:
a   lies deep to the deep fascia of the chest wall. ( )
b   extends from the side of the sternum to near
    the midaxillary line. ( )
c   has a subcutaneous and submammary plexus
    of lymph vessels. ( )

d   develops from modified skin glands. ( )

e   has a lymphatic drainage which extends to the
    anterior mediastinum. ( )

40 The adult heart:
a   is related posteriorly to the oesophagus, left
    main bronchus and aorta. ( )
b   lies on the left dome of the diaphragm. ( )

c   in health weighs approximately 900 g. ( )
d   admits the great veins on its posterior surface. ( )

e   is totally enclosed by the serous pericardium. ( )

41 The right atrium:
a   is related to the central tendon of the diaphragm
    at the level of the 8th thoracic vertebra. ( )

b   has a thin anterior endocardial fold "guarding"
    the superior vena cava. ( )
c   has an auricle situated superolaterally. ( )

d   has the coronary sinus opening situated between
    the fossa ovalis and the opening of the inferior
    vena cava. ( )
e   has a fossa ovalis on the atrioventricular wall. ( )

a F— it is a subcutaneous structure lying in the superficial fascia.
b T— And vertically from the 2nd to the 6th rib.

c T— These drain laterally to the pectoral nodes; superiorly to the infraclavicular and lower deep cervical nodes; medially to the parasternal nodes (some lymph vessels cross the midline to the nodes and the plexuses of the opposite side); and inferiorly to the anterior abdominal wall plexuses and the diaphragmatic nodes.

d T— It originates as an ectodermal downgrowth on the 'milkline' between the axilla and the groin.
e T— Lymph drains to the axilla, the deep cervical nodes and medially to the parasternal nodes and the opposite breast.

a T— The square base is separated from these structures by the pericardial sac.
b F— Inferiorly it is related to the central tendon of the diaphragm, to which the fibrous pericardium is firmly attached.
c F— 300 g is the average weight of the adult heart.
d T— The four pulmonary veins enter the left atrium posteriorly; the superior and inferior venae cavae enter the posterior part of the right atrium.
e T— The serous pericardium is a closed serous sac invaginated by the heart. It encloses a thin pericardial cavity.

a T— The inferior vena cava enters the atrium at this point. The wall of the atrium between the inferior and the superior venae cavae forms the right border of the heart.
b F— The superior vena cava has no valve. There is an anterior fold 'guarding' the entry of the inferior vena cava.
c F— The auricle lies superomedially against the beginning of the aorta. On the inner surface, a ridge (crista terminalis) separates the rough-walled auricle from the smooth-walled atrium.
d F— The sinus opening lies between the fossa ovalis and the opening into the right ventricle. The sinus opening is 'guarded' by an endocardial fold.
e F— The fossa lies on the interatrial wall, a remnant of the fetal foramen ovale.

42 **The right ventricle:**
  a forms most of the inferior surface of the heart. (   )

  b is normally oval in cross section. (   )

  c has a tricuspid valve in its inflow tract. (   )
  d usually contains three conical papillary muscles. (   )

  e possesses a pulmonary orifice guarded by a
     tricuspid valve. (   )

43 **The mitral valve:**
  a possesses two cusps. (   )

  b 'guards' the right atrioventricular orifice. (   )
  c is closely related to the aortic valve. .(   )

  d has no papillary muscle attachments. (   )

  e lies on the posterior wall of the left ventricle. (   )

44 **The coronary arteries:**
  a arise from the inferior aspect of the aortic arch. (   )

  b each gives atrial and ventricular branches. (   )
  c anastomose extensively with each other. (   )
  d supply the conducting system of the heart. (   )

  e supply the papillary muscles of the mitral and
     tricuspid valves. (   )

a T— It forms part of the anterior and most of the inferior surface of the heart.

b F— The interventricular septum bulges into its cavity making it crescentic in cross section.

c T— The tricuspid valve has fine tendinous cords anchoring its

d F cusps inferiorly. These arise from two papillary muscles and from the interventricular septum directly.

e T— The pulmonary semilunar valve possesses three semilunar valve cusps.

a T— Each cusp consists of a double fold of endocardium and a small amount of fibrous tissue. Normally it is avascular.

b F— The left atrioventricular orifice is 'guarded'.

c T— The anterior cusp is larger and lies between the aortic and mitral orifices.

d F— Both cusps are anchored by tendinous cords to papillary muscles arising from the walls of the left ventricle.

e T

a F— The right coronary artery arises from the anterior aortic sinus and the left from the left posterior sinus immediately adjacent to the aortic valve.

b T— The right artery supplies most of the right side of the heart

c T and the left supplies the left side, but, although they

d T anastomose in the septum and apex, sudden occlusion of a large branch may result in death of heart muscle. The conducting system is supplied by the coronary vessels and damage to it may have rapid catastrophic consequences.

e T— Occlusion of the coronary vessels may cause death of a papillary muscle and its rupture.

45 **The atrioventricular bundle:**
  a forms part of the conducting system of the heart. (   )

  b is formed of nervous tissue. (   )
  c lies in the interventricular septum. (   )

  d divides into two branches and then ramifies as
     the subendocardial plexus. (   )
  e bridges between the atrial and ventricular muscles. (   )

46 **During the development of the heart:**
  a the venae cavae come to enter the caudal end
     of the heart tube. (   )
  b the oblique sinus of the pericardium arises
     from the serous pericardium enveloping the major
     arteries. (   )
  c division into right and left sides is completed
     prior to birth. (   )

  d the pulmonary veins and venae cavae are
     incorporated into the walls of the left and right atria
     respectively. (   )
  e there is very little blood flow to the developing lungs. (   )

47 **The ascending aorta:**
  a ascends as far as the right sternoclavicular joint. (   )
  b lies intrapericardially. (   )

  c has no branches. (   )

  d is related posteriorly to the right main bronchus. (   )

  e is related anteriorly to the sternum. (   )

a **T**— The system comprises all of the tissues which convey electrical impulses to the cardiac muscle, viz. — the sino-atrial node, the atrioventricular node, the AV bundle, its branches and the subendocardial plexus.

b **F**— It arises from the specialised cardiac muscle cells.

c **T**— It lies in the membranous interventricular septum and divides into right and left ventricular branches.

d **T**— On the ventricular wall the subendocardial plexus consists of the Purkinje fibres.

e **T**— The AV bundle is the only continuity between the atria and ventricles, whose muscles are separated by a pair of fibrous rings encircling both atrioventricular valves.

a **T**— Bending of the heart tube occurs and the precursors of these vessels then enter posteriorly.

b **F**— This cul-de-sac is formed by the pericardial reflection around the pulmonary veins and inferior vena cava.

c **F**— During intra-uterine life the foramen ovale remains patent allowing oxygenated placental blood to flow from the right to the left atrium and bypass the 'functionless' lungs. The foramen usually closes at birth or soon after.

d **T**— Forming the smooth posterior part of their walls.

e **T**— The patent foramen ovale and the ductus venosus, between the pulmonary artery and aorta, ensure most blood bypasses the fetal lung.

a **F**— It is 5 cm long, ending at the level of the sternal angle.

b **T**— Within the fibrous pericardium enclosed in a sheath of serous pericardium common to it and the pulmonary artery.

c **F**— The right and left coronary arteries arise near its origin from the anterior and left posterior aortic sinuses respectively.

d **T**— And, inferior to this, to the right pulmonary artery and the left atrium.

e **T**— The sternum lies directly adjacent.

48   The arch of the aorta:

a   arches posteriorly over the root of the right lung.   (   )

b   is related, on its left side, to mediastinal pleura.   (   )

c   is connected to the right pulmonary artery.   (   )

d   is related to the left brachiocephalic vein superiorly.   (   )

e   is related anteriorly to the manubrium sternum.   (   )

49   The descending thoracic aorta:

a   ends on the front of the 12th thoracic vertebra.   (   )

b   is directly related to both the left and right pleura.   (   )

c   gives branches to the bronchi.   (   )

d   is related anteriorly to the pulmonary trunk.   (   )

e   has the thoracic duct on its left side.   (   )

50   The pulmonary trunk:

a   lies at its origin anterior to the root of the aorta.   (   )

b   is contained within a common sleeve of
serous pericardium with the ascending aorta.   (   )

c   bifurcates anterior to the aortic arch.   (   )

d   is related to the left pleura and lung.   (   )

e   is closely related to both right and left
coronary arteries.   (   )

a F— It arches posteriorly over the root of the left lung and reaches the left side of the 4th thoracic vertebra.

b T— Which separates it from the left lung. The left phrenic and vagus nerves lie on its left side.

c F— There is a fibrous connection to the left pulmonary artery — the ligamentum arteriosum, a fibrous remnant of the ductus arteriosus.

d T— As the vein crosses obliquely above the aortic arch. The brachiocephalic, left common carotid and left subclavian branches of the aorta lie behind the vein.

e T— The arch commences at the sternomanubrial junction and lies directly behind the manubrium.

a T— It descends from the left side of the 4th thoracic vertebra and inclines medially, passes through the diaphragm at the level of the 12th thoracic vertebra and becomes the abdominal aorta.

b T— Throughout its course it is in contact with the left pleura and inferiorly the oesophagus leaves its right side so that it is then directly related to the right pleura and lung.

c T— Two or three such vessels arise, together with posterior intercostal, subcostal, oesophageal and diaphragmatic branches.

d F— Its anterior relations from above downwards are the root of the left lung, the oesophagus and the diaphragm.

e F— The duct lies alongside the azygos vein to the right of the aorta.

a T— Then it ascends posteriorly and to the left.

b T— All contained within the fibrous pericardium.

c F— It bifurcates posterior to and to the left of the aorta within the concavity of the aortic arch.

d T— Both its anterior and left surfaces are related to the left pleura and lung.

e T— These vessels surround its base.

51   The brachiocephalic vein:

a   of both right and left sides is formed by the
     union of the internal jugular and subclavian veins.   (   )
b   enters the right atrium directly.   (   )

c   on the right side is related to the right pleura.   (   )
d   on the right is related to the thoracic duct.   (   )

e   on the left, gains tributaries from the thyroid gland.   (   )

52   The azygos vein:

a   originates in the abdomen.   (   )

b   leaves the abdomen by the oesophageal opening.   (   )
c   drains into the right atrium directly.   (   )

d   receives both right bronchial and right posterior
     intercostal tributaries.   (   )

e   receives small pulmonary tributaries.   (   )

53   The left phrenic nerve:

a   arises from the dorsal rami of the 3rd, 4th and 5th
     cervical nerves.   (   )

b   descends through the thorax in the left pleural cavity.   (   )

c   receives sensory branches from the mediastinal
     and diaphragmatic pleura and from the
     diaphragmatic peritoneum.   (   )
d   passes through the caval opening of the diaphragm.   (   )

e   descends in the thorax posterior to the lung root.   (   )

a **T**— This occurs behind the respective sternoclavicular joint.

b **F**— The two veins unite behind the right border of the manubrium and form the superior vena cava.

c **T**— Separated from it only by the right phrenic nerve.

d **F**— The thoracic duct enters the origin of the left vein, a smaller right lymph duct often enters the origin of the right vein.

e **T**— Inferior thyroid veins unite to enter the left brachiocephalic vein.

a **T**— Usually by the union of the right subcostal and right ascending lumbar veins. On the left side the accessory hemiazygos is formed.

b **F**— It leaves through the aortic opening.

c **F**— It arches over the root of the right lung at the level of the 4th thoracic vertebra and enters the superior vena cava.

d **T**— The left intercostal and bronchial veins drain via the hemi-azygos and accessory hemiazygos veins into the azygos vein.

e **F**— Venous blood from the lung parenchyma drains into the pulmonary veins.

a **F**— It arises from the ventral rami of these nerves, descends on the anterior surface of scalenus anterior and passes through the thoracic inlet.

b **F**— It has a long mediastinal course and is covered by the left mediastinal pleura.

c **T**— And gives motor branches to the diaphragm.

d **F**— The left phrenic nerve pierces the dome of the diaphragm, sending branches to its undersurface. The right phrenic nerve passes through the caval opening of the diaphragm.

e **F**— Both phrenic nerves lie anterior to the lung root.

54   **The right vagus nerve during its course in the thorax:**

a   lies posterolateral to the right brachiocephalic artery. (   )

b   is separated from the mediastinal pleura by the trachea.   (   )

c   contributes to the pulmonary plexus.   (   )

d   contributes to the oesophageal plexus.   (   )

e   gives off the right recurrent laryngeal nerve.   (   )

55   **The gastric nerves:**

a   both arise from the oesophageal plexus.   (   )

b   contain only fibres from the right and left vagi.   (   )

c   supply branches to the liver.   (   )

d   supply branches to the coeliac plexus.   (   )

e   supply branches to the pancreas.   (   )

56   **The thymus:**

a   is a glandular structure which normally atrophies shortly after birth.   (   )

b   lies posterior to the trachea.   (   )

c   contains large numbers of lymphocytes.   (   )

d   is derived from the fourth pair of pharnygeal pouches.   (   )

e   is derived from thyroid tissue.   (   )

a T— As it descends in the thorax posterolateral to the
b F brachiocephalic artery it lies between the trachea and
     mediastinal pleura.
c T— It gives branches to the pulmonary plexus before
d T terminating with branches of the left vagus in the
     oesophageal plexus.
e F— This branch arises in the neck and loops upward around
     the right subclavian artery.

a T— Both anterior and posterior gastric nerves arise from the
     oesophageal plexus and contain both vagal and
b F sympathetic fibres.
c T— After descending through the diaphragm the anterior nerve
d T supplies the stomach, duodenum, pancreas and liver. The
e T posterior nerve supplies the stomach and branches to the
     coeliac plexus.

a F— It is large at birth, but normally atrophies before puberty.

b F— It lies in front of the trachea at the root of the neck. It is
     variable in size and may extend down, in front of the aortic
     arch and its branches, into the mediastinum.

c T— It is a lobulated structure with a cortex in which
     lymphocytes are predominant and a medulla which
     contains thymocytes and concentrically arranged cells —
     Hassall's corpuscles.

d F— It is derived from the third pair of pharyngeal pouches.

e F

57 **The thoracic oesophagus:**
a lies posterior to the trachea. ( )

b is directly related to the vertebral column
throughout its course. ( )

c is related to the left atrium. ( )
d pierces the central tendon of the diaphragm at
the level of the 8th thoracic vertebra. ( )

e is crossed by the left bronchus. ( )

58 **The thoracic trachea:**
a bifurcates at the level of the sternal angle. ( )

b is closely related to the azygos vein. ( )

c has complete fibrocartilaginous rings within its
walls. ( )

d is related anteriorly to the thyroid gland. ( )

e ends at the level of the sternal angle. ( )

59 **The right extrapulmonary bronchus:**
a is longer than the left. ( )
b lies more vertically than the left. ( )

c lies posterior to the pulmonary artery. ( )

d lies posterior to the pulmonary veins. ( )

e lies below the arch of the azygos vein. ( )

a **T**— With the left recurrent laryngeal nerve and the right vagus lying in the grooves between it and the trachea.

b **F**— Superiorly this is so, but inferiorly it is separated from the vertebral column by the thoracic duct, the azygos and accessory hemiazygos veins, the right posterior intercostal arteries and the thoracic aorta.

c **T**— Separated only by the pericardium of the oblique sinus.

d **F**— The oesophageal opening is surrounded by muscular fibres from the right crus of the diaphragm, and is found to the left of the midline at the level of the 10th thoracic vertebra.

e **T**— The left bronchus crosses the middle third of the oesophagus anteriorly.

a **T**— The bifurcation is at this level and that of the 4th thoracic vertebra, and lies to the right of and behind the pulmonary trunk bifurcation.

b **T**— In its lower part it is separated from the mediastinal pleura by the azygos vein.

c **F**— Its walls are formed of a fibrous skeleton strengthened by 15–20 incomplete hyaline cartilage rings (plates) and smooth muscle.

d **F**— The thymus is found in front of the trachea in a child and thymic remnants in the adult. The thyroid gland is in the neck.

e **T**— Its bifurcation, the carina is at this level and that of the 4th thoracic vertebra.

a **F**— The right bronchus is shorter but wider than the left.

b **T**— Inhaled foreign material more easily enters the right bronchus.

c **T**— The bifurcation of the pulmonary trunk occurs at the same level as the bifurcation of the trachea and results in both right and left pulmonary arteries lying anterior to the main bronchi.

d **T**— The pulmonary veins lie inferior to both the bronchus and the artery on both sides.

e **T**— The azygos vein ascends behind the right bronchus to enter the superior vena cava.

60   The surface markings of the pleural sacs:
   a   do not extend above the clavicle.   (   )
   b   are similar on the right and left sides.   (·   )
   c   meet in the midline anteriorly.   (   )
   d   extend to the 8th rib in the midaxillary line. (   )

   e   extend to the 12th rib in the paravertebral line. (   )

61   The right lung:
   a   is larger than the left.   (   )

   b   is divided by fissures into the upper and lower
       lobes and the lingula.   (   )

   c   possesses 10 bronchopulmonary segments.   (   )

   d   is related to the oesophagus only in the lower
       part of its medial surface.   (   )

   e   is related inferiorly to the liver.   (   )

a F— On both sides the upper limit of the pleura sacs lies 3 cm
b F above the middle of the medial third of the clavicle. The
c T pleura meet in the midline at the level of the 2nd costal
d F cartilage. At the 4th costal cartilage the left pleura
deviates laterally and descends along the lateral border of
the sternum to the 6th cartilage. Whereas the right pleura
decends vertically close to the midline to this level. They
then both deviate laterally and reach the 8th rib in the
midclavicular line and the 10th rib in the midaxillary line.
e T— The pleural reflection on to the diaphragm often lies just
inferior to the 12th rib and lateral to the paravertebral line.

a T— The right weighs about 620 g and the left about 560 g.
(The heart has to be accommodated on the left side.)
b F— The oblique and horizontal fissures divide it into upper,
middle and lower lobes. The lingula is the thin antero-
inferior portion of the left upper lobe representing the
middle lobe of the left lung.
c T— The bronchopulmonary segments are functionally
independent units of lung tissue. In the right lung there are
three in the upper lobe, two in the middle and five in the
lower lobe. The left lung is divided into five upper and five
lower segments.
d F— The medial surface of the right lung is related to the
oesophagus throughout its thoracic course except where
the azygos vein crosses over the hilus of the lung.
e T— And is separated from it by the right dome of the
diaphragm.

62 The lung tissue:

a receives its oxygenated arterial supply via branches of the thoracic aorta. ( )

b has venous drainage into the azygos system of veins. ( )

c has no lymph drainage. ( )

d has ciliated columnar epithelial lining throughout. ( )

e receives a nerve supply from the vagus. ( )

63 The thoracic sympathetic trunk:

a possesses 11 ganglia. ( )

b lies in front of the necks of the ribs. ( )

c has no direct communication with the lumbar sympathetic trunk. ( )

d provides the greater and lesser splanchnic and least splanchnic (renal) nerves. ( )

e is independent of the thoracic spinal nerves. ( )

64 Thoracic lymph vessels:

a lying in the chest wall drain to axillary lymph nodes. ( )

b in the lungs drain to tracheobronchial nodes. ( )

c drain from the oesophagus to posterior mediastinal nodes. ( )

d do not communicate with those draining the abdominal contents. ( )

e all drain into the thoracic and right lymph duct. ( )

a **T**— The bronchial arteries arise from the descending thoracic aorta.

b **T**— Bronchial veins drain to the azygos and hemiazygos veins.

c **F**— There is a rich subpleural lymph plexus, and a deep lymph plexus accompanying the bronchi. They drain via hilar and tracheobronchial nodes to mediastinal lymph trunks.

d **F**— Ciliated columnar epithelium lines the extra- and the intra-pulmonary bronchi. The terminal respiratory bronchioles are however lined by nonciliated columnar (cubical) epithelium and the alveoli by squamous epithelium.

e **T**— As vagal branches pass through the pulmonary plexus they produce bronchoconstriction.

a **F**— It usually possesses 12 ganglia, one corresponding to each thoracic nerve.

b **T**— It lies alongside the vertebral column on the necks of the ribs.

c **F**— It is continuous above with the cervical (through the thoracic inlet), and below with the lumbar sympathetic trunk (below the medial arcuate ligament).

d **T**— The greater arises from the 5th–9th ganglia, the lesser from the 9th–10th and the least (renal) from the 11th. They descend the posterior thoracic wall, pierce the crura of the diaphragm and give branches to the coeliac and pre-aortic plexuses.

e **F**— Two rami communicantes pass to each spinal nerve.

a **T**— Lymphatics drain from the superficial layers of the chest wall to the axillary nodes and from the deeper layers to parasternal and intercostal nodes.

b **T**— The thoracic viscera drain to three sets of nodes; anterior
c **T**   mediastinal, tracheobronchial and posterior mediastinal.

d **F**— Those vessels draining from the diaphragmatic nodes pass through the diaphragm to communicate with vessels draining the upper surface of the liver.

e **T** – The thoracic duct drains the left half of the chest viscera and the right lymph duct, when present, drains the right sided viscera.

65 **The thoracic duct:**

a   arises in the thorax.   ( )

b   ascends anterior to the vertebral column.   ( )
c   drains into the left brachiocephalic vein.   ( )

d   drains mainly thoracic structures.   ( )

e   is joined by the right lymph duct.   ( )

IV   Abdomen

66   **The lateral muscles of the anterior abdominal wall are:**

a   supplied by the lower six thoracic nerves and
the first lumbar nerve.   ( )

b   contained within the rectus sheath.   ( )

c   attached to the lateral margin of rectus abdominis.   ( )

d   attached in part to the costal cartilages.   ( )

e   each gain attachment to the pubic bone.   ( )

a **F**— It arises in the abdomen from the cisterna chyli and enters the thorax through the aortic opening of the diaphragm.

b **T**— Behind the oesophagus, to the left of the azygos vein.

c **T**— It arches forwards from behind the carotid sheath, anterior to the subclavian artery and enters the vein.

d **F**— It drains all the body below the diaphragm, and the left half of the body above the diaphragm through left mediastinal, jugular and subclavian lymph trunks.

e **F**— The right lymph duct is often absent but, when present, it enters the right brachiocephalic vein, draining lymph from the right side of the head, neck and thorax.

a **T**— The nerves mainly lie between the internal oblique and the transversus abdominis. Terminal branches pierce the rectus sheath and supply the rectus abdominis. Skin and peritoneum are also supplied.

b **F**— The rectus sheath of each side is formed by the aponeuroses of the three lateral muscles. The sheaths join in the midline to form a strong midline raphe.

c **F**— The aponeurosis of the internal oblique splits to enclose rectus abdominis in the umbilical region. The sheath is reinforced anteriorly by external oblique, and posteriorly by transversus abdominis.

d **T**— Both external oblique and transversus abdominis originate by fleshy muscle fibres from the outer and inner aspects respectively of the lower six ribs and costal cartilages. Internal oblique is attached laterally to the costal margin.

e **T**— Internal oblique and transversus by the conjoint tendon and external oblique by the inguinal ligament.

67   The inguinal canal:

a   extends between a defect in the transversalis fascia
and a defect in the external oblique aponeurosis.   (   )

b   has an anterior wall comprising the external
oblique aponeurosis and the internal oblique
muscle.   (   )

c   has its floor formed by the deep fascia of the thigh.   (   )

d   has its posterior wall formed medially by
peritoneum.   (   )

e   is longer in the newborn than the adult.   (   )

68   The spermatic cord:

a   has three fascial coverings.   (   )

b   contains three arteries.   (   )

c   contains three nerves.   (   )

d   contains one muscle.   (   )

e   is less well developed in the female.   (   )

a T—The deep inguinal ring is a defect in transversalis fascia laterally and the superficial inguinal ring a defect in the external oblique aponeurosis medially.

b T—The internal oblique reinforces the lateral part of the anterior wall. The internal oblique fibres arch over the cord, join with the transversus abdominis fibres and form the conjoint tendon.

c F—The floor is the upper surface of the inguinal ligament which is continuous with the deep fascia of the thigh and the aponeurosis of the external oblique.

d F—The posterior wall is formed by peritoneum and fascia transversalis. They are reinforced medially by the conjoint tendon, i.e. behind the superficial inguinal ring.

e F—In the newborn, the external ring lies almost directly over the internal ring; it is therefore shorter and less oblique than in the adult.

a T—The internal spermatic fascia is continuous with the transversalis fascia, the cremasteric fascia and muscle are continuous with the internal oblique, and the external spermatic fascia is continuous with the external oblique.

b T—The testicular, cremasteric and the artery to the ductus deferens.

c T—The genital branch of the genitofemoral nerve, the ilioinguinal nerve and sympathetic nerves.

d T—The cremasteric muscle which mediates the cremasteric reflex. The testis is drawn up when the skin of the medial side of the thigh is stimulated.

e T—The spermatic cord is formed as the testis descends through the inguinal canal into the scrotum. It is absent in the female.

69   The testis:
a   has the epididymus applied to its medial side.   (   )

b   is supplied by sympathetic nerves originating
in the 10th thoracic segment.   (   )

c   is drained by lymph vessels passing to the external
iliac lymph nodes.   (   )
d   descends into the scrotum just before birth.   (   )

e   is covered in the scrotum by one layer of fascia.   (   )

70   The testis, in its embryological development:
a   originates from coelomic mesothelium adjacent
to the mesonephros.   (   )
b   gains contributions from the developing
mesonephros.   (   )
c   is aided in its descent by the processus vaginalis.   (   )

d   does not normally complete its descent into the
scrotum until three months after birth.   (   )
e   causes inguinal hernias to be more common
in the male.   (   )

71   The lesser omentum:
a   is attached superiorly to the porta hepatis and
the fissure for the ligamentum venosum.   (   )

b   extends inferiorly as far as the transverse colon.   (   )

c   separates the lesser sac (omental bursa) and
greater sac of peritoneum.   (   )

d   forms part of the boundaries of the epiploic
foramen.   (   )
e   embraces the portal vein.   (   )

46

a   **F**— The epididymis is applied to its posterolateral aspect and is connected to the testis by about 20 deferent ducts.

b   **T**— This is the consequence of its development from the coelomic mesothelium of the upper posterior abdominal wall. The corresponding dermatome includes the umbilicus.

c   **F**— Drainage is to the para-aortic nodes in the region of the renal vessels.

d   **T**— It descends the posterior abdominal wall and then the inguinal canal, preceded by the gubernaculum, prior to birth. It takes a covering of peritoneum, the processus vaginalis, with it. This becomes the tunica vaginalis.

e   **F**— It is covered by four layers. From within outwards, the internal spermatic fascia, cremasteric fascia, external spermatic fascia and superficial fascia containing the dartos muscle.

a   **T**— It develops from the coelomic mesothelium of the posterior abdominal wall. Tubules of the mesonephros

b   **T** become the efferent ducts and the head of the epididymis. The mesonephric duct becomes the ductus deferens.

c   **F**— Testicular descent is aided by the gubernaculum, a mesodermal mass attached to its lower pole. Descent into

d   **F** the scrotum is usually complete at birth.

e   **T**— The processus vaginalis may result in inguinal hernias appearing any time from birth onwards.

a   **T**— Its 2 layers are formed from the left and right sacs of peritoneum covering the liver which meet along this line. The falciform ligament, formed in a similar way, passes from the liver to the anterior abdominal wall above the umbilicus. The ligament and lesser omentum are both remnants of the fetal ventral mesentery.

b   **F**— It passes inferiorly, meets and encloses from above downwards the oesophagus, stomach and initial part of the duodenum.

c   **T**— The lesser sac lies behind the lesser omentum and stomach, and communicates with the greater sac only by the epiploic foramen.

d   **T**— This foramen is bounded anteriorly by the free edge of the lesser omentum, superiorly by the liver, posteriorly by the

e   **T** inferior vena cava and inferiorly by the duodenum. The free edge contains the bile duct, hepatic artery and the portal vein.

72   The mesentery:

a   of the small intestine is attached obliquely along a line extending from the descending part of the duodenum to the left sacro-iliac joint.   (   )

b   of the small intestine contains branches of the inferior mesenteric artery.   (   )

c   of the transverse colon is attached horizontally to the anterior border of the pancreas.   (·   )

d   of the sigmoid colon lies over the promontory of the sacrum.   (   )

e   of the sigmoid colon contains the inferior mesenteric vein.   (   )

73   The pelvic peritoneum:

a   covers both the uterus and uterine tubes.   (   )

b   condenses and forms the round ligaments of the uterus.   (   )

c   covers the anterior surface of the rectum only in its upper third.   (   )

d   covers the superior surface of the bladder in both sexes.   (   )

e   can be palpated by means of a digital examination of the rectum.   (   )

74   The abdominal oesophagus:

a   enters the abdomen between the right and left crus of the diaphragm.   (   )

b   is enveloped by peritoneum.   (   )

c   is closely related to both the anterior and posterior gastric nerves.   (   )

d   is closely related to the left lobe of the liver.   (   )

e   is surrounded by an external oesophageal sphincter. (   )

a F— Its oblique attachment extends from the duodenojejunal flexure (on the left side of L2 vertebra) to the ileocolic junction (overlying the right sacro-iliac joint).

b F— The arteries it contains are branches of the superior mesenteric artery which supplies derivatives of the midgut.

c T— Its horizontal attachment extends to the left across the descending part of the duodenum, the anterior border of the pancreas and the tail of the pancreas as it crosses the anterior surface of the left kidney.

d F— The sigmoid mesocolon is attached on the posterior pelvic wall along a ∧-shaped line whose apex lies over the left sacro-iliac joint.

e T— Conveying the vein to the posterior abdominal wall where it ascends to join the splenic vein.

a T— It covers anterior and posterior surfaces of the uterus and the tubes, and extends to the pelvic walls forming the broad ligaments of the uterus.

b F— The round ligaments of the uterus are remnants of the gubernaculum of the ovary.

c F— Anteriorly the rectum is covered by peritoneum in its upper two-thirds.

d T— And extends over the upper part of its posterior surface. In the male, the upper part of the seminal vesicles are also covered.

e T— The rectovaginal, or in the male the rectovesical, pouch of peritoneum can be palpated in this manner through the rectal wall. Pelvic peritonitis may thus be diagnosed.

a F— The oesophageal opening of the diaphragm lies within the fibres of the right crus to the left of the midline.

b F— Peritoneum covers only its anterior surface.

c T— The anterior gastric nerve is often within its wall and the posterior gastric nerve is adjacent to its posterior surface.

d T— It lies between the diaphragm posteriorly and the left lobe of the liver anteriorly.

e F— The lower oesophageal sphincter lies within the oesophageal wall. Competence of the sphincter is aided by the oblique angle of entry of the oesophagus into the stomach.

75 **In the stomach, the:**

a fundus lies above the level of the oesophageal opening. (   )

b body extends inferiorly to the angular notch. (   )

c right border is known as its greater curvature. (   )

d cardiac orifice is closely related to the aorta. (   )

e blood supply arises from midgut arteries. (   )

76 **The stomach:**

a is supplied in part by arteries arising from the splenic artery. (   )

b is supplied by arteries which each arise from branches of the coeliac trunk. (   )

c has a venous drainage passing equally to the portal and systemic venous systems. (   )

d is lined by columnar and squamous epithelium. (   )

e is totally covered by serosa (peritoneum). (   )

77 **The duodenum:**

a is almost completely covered by peritoneum. (   )

b lies behind the portal vein. (   )

c lies anterior to the hilus of the right kidney. (   )

d is crossed anteriorly by the superior mesenteric vessels. (   )

e is about 25 cm long. (   )

a **T**— The fundus is that part lying above the oesophageal opening.

b **T**— The body extends from the fundus to the angular notch, the lowest point of the lesser curvature.

c **F**— The greater curvature is the left border extending from the left of the oesophagus around the fundus and body to the pylorus.

d **F**— The cardiac orifice and the oesophagus lie between the diaphragm and the liver and are separated from the aorta by fibres from the right crus of the diaphragm.

e **F**— The blood supply is by the short gastric arteries, the right and left gastric arteries, and the right and left gastro-epiploic arteries; all of these are branches of the coeliac, a foregut artery.

a **T**— The short gastric vessels, supplying the fundus and the left gastro-epiploic, supplying most of the greater curvature, arise from the splenic.

b **T**— The left and right gastric, the left and right gastro-epiploic and the short gastric arteries each arise from branches of the coeliac trunk or the trunk itself.

c **F**— All blood from the stomach normally passes to the portal vein. There are, however, anastomoses with oesophageal veins.

d **F**— It is lined completely by columnar epithelium and contains three different types of glands. The cardiac glands secrete mucus only; the acid and enzyme secreting gastric glands are found largely in the body; and the pyloric glands in the antrum produce mucous and the hormone gastrin.

e **T**— Peritoneum invests the whole stomach, being reflected from it along the lines of the greater and lesser omentum, on its greater and lesser curvatures.

a **F**— Only its first and last centimetres are invested by peritoneum. The remainder lies retroperitoneally, only its anterior surface being covered.

b **F**— The ascending part of the duodenum is anterior to the portal vein, bile duct and gastroduodenal artery.

c **T**— Its descending part lies anterior to the right suprarenal, the hilus of the right kidney and the right psoas muscle.

d **T**— The root of the mesentery and the superior mesenteric vessels cross anterior to the horizontal part.

e **T**— It comprises the 1st part (5 cm), 2nd (8 cm), descending on the right of the vertebral column, 3rd (10 cm), running horizontally and the 4th part (3 cm), which ascends on the left side of the 2nd lumbar vertebra.

78   **In the small intestine the:**
a   duodenojejunal flexure lies on the left of the first
lumbar vertebra.   (   )
b   jejunum has a thicker wall than the ileum.   (   )

c   arterial arcades are less numerous in the jejunum
than in the ileum.   (   )
d   root of the mesentery crosses the left psoas muscle. (   )

e   jejunum lies above and to the left of the ileum.   (   )

79   **The caecum:**
a   is completely invested in peritoneum.   (   )
b   possesses a longitudinal muscle coat but no
taeniae coli.   (   )
c   lies on the right psoas muscle.   (   )

d   has an ileocaecal orifice opening inferiorly.   (   )
e   lies adjacent to the right femoral nerve.   (   )

80   **The appendix:**
a   arises from the inferior aspect of the caecum.   (

b   has a mesentery.   (

c   is commonly absent.   (
d   usually lies retrocaecally.   (

e   is clothed in peritoneum.   (

a **F**— The root of the mesentery passes from the left side of the 2nd lumbar vertebra to the right sacro-iliac joint.

b **T**— The jejunum is also wider. Its mucous membrane is thrown into circular folds with many villi but there are fewer aggregations of lymphoid tissue in the wall and less fat in the mesentery than in the ileum.

c **T**— The jejunal vessels are larger, and the jejunal wall is more vascular than the ileal.

d **T**— It then crosses in turn the aorta, inferior vena cava, right gonadal vessels, right ureter and right psoas muscle.

e **T**

a **T**— It does not generally possess a mesentery.

b **F**— The longitudinal muscle is arranged in three bands, the taeniae coli, which converge on to the appendix.

c **T**— It lies anterior to the iliacus and psoas muscles in the right iliac fossa.

d **F**— The ileocaecal orifice opens to its medial wall.

e **T**— The femoral nerve and the external iliac vessels lie on its medial side.

a **F**— It arises from the posteromedial wall of the caecum 3 cm below the ileocaecal orifice.

b **T**— Its peritoneal coat extends and forms its mesentery which connects it to the terminal ileum.

c **F**— Absence of the appendix is extremely rare.

d **T**— Though its mobility leads to great variation in its position, it most commonly lies retrocaecally.

e **T**— This peritoneum is reflected from the appendix to form the mesoappendix.

81   The sigmoid colon:

a   extends from the pelvic brim to the third sacral
segment.   (   )

b   is closely tethered by its peritoneal covering.   (   )
c   lies in close proximity to both ureters.   (   )

d   lies adjacent to the bladder in both sexes.   (   )
e   is supplied by branches of the inferior mesenteric
artery.   (   )

82   The coeliac trunk:

a   arises at the level of the inferior border of the pancreas. (   )
b   has three main branches.   (   )

c   is surrounded by a plexus of nerves.   (   )
d   supplies the foregut and structures derived from it.   (   )

e   supplies the lower oesophagus.   (   )

83   The splenic artery:

a   reaches the hilus of the spleen by a retroperitoneal
course.   (   )
b   lies aiong the upper border of the pancreas.   (   )
c   supplies branches to the stomach.   (   )

d   supplies branches to the left adrenal gland.   (   )
e   lies anterior to the left kidney.   (   )

84   The superior mesenteric artery:

a   arises behind the body of the pancreas.   (   )
b   supplies no bowel proximal to the duodenojejunal
flexure.   (   )
c   supplies the bowel as far as the left side of the
transverse colon.   (   )
d   ends by dividing into ileocolic and right colic vessels. (   )

e   lies posterior to the uncinate process.   (   )

a **T**— At the third sacral segment it becomes continuous with the rectum. Its position is variable for it is attached by a mesentery to the pelvic wall.

b **F**

c **F**— Posteriorly it lies on the left ureter and is related inferiorly in both sexes to the bladder.

d **T**

e **T**— Sigmoid arterial branches enter the sigmoid mesocolon to supply the structure.

a **F**— It arises from the aorta just above the pancreas.

b **T**— After passing forward for 2 cm it divides into the left gastric, common hepatic and splenic arteries.

c **T**— These nerves and ganglia form the coeliac (solar) plexus.

d **T**— The coeliac trunk supplies the foregut, the superior mesenteric the midgut, and the inferior mesenteric the hindgut structures.

e **T**— Oesophageal branches of the left gastric artery supply the lower third of the oesophagus.

a **F**— Its initial tortuous course along the upper border of the pancreas is retroperitoneal, but it reaches the hilus of the spleen by passing in the lienorenal ligament.

b **T**

c **T**— Its short gastric branches pass to the fundus of the stomach in the gastrosplenic ligament and its left gastro-epiploic branch passes to the greater curvature of the stomach.

d **F**— Its only other branches are several pancreatic branches.

e **T**— In addition, it is anterior to the left crus of the diaphragm and left psoas muscle.

a **T**— Its origin from the aorta is behind the body of the pancreas.

b **F**— The inferior pancreaticoduodenal artery supplies the lower duodenum as far as the duodenal papilla and also the pancreas.

c **T**— At this point its branch, the middle colic artery, anastomoses with the left colic, a branch of the inferior mesenteric artery.

d **T**— After giving 15–20 jejunal and ileal branches it ends in the right iliac fossa by dividing into these branches.

e **F**— It descends behind the body of the pancreas to emerge anterior to the uncinate process after which it gains the small bowel mesentery.

85   The inferior mesenteric artery:

a   supplies the large bowel from the left part of the
transverse colon to the upper anal canal.   (   )

b   continues as the inferior rectal artery in the pelvis.   (   )

c   anastomoses with branches of the internal iliac
artery.   (   )

d   is crossed over by the left ureter.   (   )

e   contributes to the marginal artery of the bowel.   (   )

86   The portal vein:

a   drains venous blood from the whole of the
intra-abdominal alimentary tract.   (   )

b   receives the splenic vein as a tributary.   (   )

c   receives branches from the liver.   (   )

d   is closely related to the bile duct and common
hepatic artery.   (   )

e   gains tributaries from the anterior abdominal wall. .   (   )

87   The splenic vein:

a   lies posterior to the pancreas.   (   )

b   unites with the superior mesenteric vein.   (   )

c   has tributaries draining into it from the stomach.   (   )

d   drains into the systemic venous system.   (   )

e   has the inferior mesenteric vein as a tributary.   (   )

a **T**— It supplies this distal part of the large bowel and upper anal canal by the left colic and sigmoid arteries, and by its continuation in the pelvis, the superior rectal artery.

b **F**— The inferior rectal artery is a branch of the internal pudendal artery.

c **T**— Its terminal branch, the superior rectal artery, anastomoses with the inferior rectal branch of the internal pudendal artery in the wall of the anal canal.

d **F**— The artery descends on the posterior abdominal wall with the left ureter on its left side, separated from it by the inferior mesenteric vein. The branches cross over the ureter.

e **T**— Ileal and colic branches of the superior and inferior mesenteric arteries form a continuous anastomotic arcade along the mesenteric border of the bowel.

a **T**— The venous drainage from all the alimentary tract, from the lower oesophagus to the upper anal canal and including the spleen, pancreas and gall bladder is into the portal vein which is formed by the junction of the splenic and superior mesenteric veins. Blood then drains along the portal vein into the liver.

b **T**

c **F**— Hepatic veins drain into the inferior vena cava.

d **T**— The portal vein ascends in the free edge of the lesser omentum behind the common hepatic artery on the left and the bile duct on the right. The vein is separated from the inferior vena cava by the epiploic foramen.

e **T**— These, the para-umbilical veins, anastomose with other veins of the abdominal wall to form a portosystemic anastomosis. When portal pressure is high the distended veins of the anastomosis are readily visible around the umbilicus — the caput medusa.

a **T**— It is formed in the hilus of the spleen by the union of tributaries from that organ, the left gastro-epiploic and short gastric veins. It passes to the right lying behind the pancreas.

b **T**

c **T**

d **F**— It unites with the superior mesenteric vein behind the neck (head) of the pancreas and forms the portal vein which drains to the liver.

e **T**— It enters the splenic vein behind the body of the pancreas.

88 **A portal-systemic anastomosis occurs between the:**
  a azygos and left gastric veins. ( )
  b epigastric veins and the veins in the falciform ( )
     ligament.

  c portal vein and the inferior vena cava. ( )
  d portal vein and renal vein. ( )
  e portal vein and the extra hepatic tributaries of the ( )
     hepatic vein.

89 **The mucous membrane of the small and large bowel
    possesses:** ( )
  a numerous lymph nodules. ( )
  b a layer of smooth muscle.

  c columnar epithelium throughout its length. ( )
  d a nerve plexus throughout its length. ( )
  e secretory cells throughout its length. ( )

90 **The liver:**
  a is attached to the diaphragm and anterior
     abdominal wall by the ligamentum venosum. ( )

  b is totally covered by peritoneum. ( )

  c is divided on the visceral surface into two lobes
     by the interlobar fissure. ( )
  d has a fibrous capsule. ( )

  e has an embryological remnant connecting it to the ( )
     umbilicus.

a T— The portal venous system anastomoses with the systemic
b T venous system at both of these sites and others which are
the 'junctional' regions such as the recto-anal junction, and
the bare areas of the gut, liver and pancreas.

c F— Neither the inferior vena cava nor renal vein have any
d F connection with the portal venous system.

e F— There is no connection between the portal vein and these
tributaries.

a T— Collections of lymph tissue occur throughout its length.

b T— The mucous membrane is divided by the muscularis
mucosae, a layer of smooth muscle.

c T— The epithelial lining contains many goblet cells.

d T— The submucous (Meissner's) nerve plexus.

e T— Mucosal cells produce mucus throughout; in addition, the
small bowel mucosa secretes hormones such as gastrin
and secretin.

a F— This liver attachment is by a fold of peritoneum, the
falciform ligament, extending from the anterior and
superior surfaces of the liver to the diaphragm and anterior
abdominal wall, and by the peritoneum bounding the bare
area of the liver, and probably most important, by the
inferior vena cava.

b F— Although largely covered by peritoneum the two layers of
the coronary ligaments diverge to enclose a part of the
diaphragmatic surface posteriorly which is bare of
peritoneum.

c T— Containing the ligamentum venosum and the ligamentum
teres.

d T— This is invaginated at the porta hepatis by the triad of
portal vein, common hepatic artery and hepatic duct and
forms a sheath around these structures in their intrahepatic
course.

e T— The ligamentum teres is the obliterated left umbilical vein
draining from the umbilicus to the left branch of the portal
vein.

91 **The liver:**
   a   drains by hepatic veins into the inferior vena cava.   (   )

   b   has a lymph drainage to both the mediastinal and porta hepatis nodes.   (   )

   c   is supplied by the phrenic nerves.   (   )

   d   is directly related to the right suprarenal gland.   (   )

   e   gains an arterial supply from the coeliac axis.   (   )

92 **The bile duct:**
   a   enters the duodenum 10 cm beyond the pylorus.   (   )

   b   lies between the portal vein and duodenum.   (   )

   c   lies anterior to the inferior vena cava in part of its course.   (   )

   d   usually has an opening into the duodenum separate from the main pancreatic duct.   (   )

   e   receives the right and left hepatic ducts.   (   )

93 **The gall bladder:**
   a   lies adjacent to the tip of the 10th right costal cartilage.   (   )

   b   is closely related to the duodenum.   (   )

   c   is supplied by a branch of the right hepatic artery.   (   )

   d   is lined by squamous epithelium.   (   )

   e   is usually completely covered with peritoneum.   (   )

a **T**— There are usually large right and left hepatic veins and several smaller branches draining blood from the liver directly into the inferior vena cava.

b **T**— The superficial (subperitoneal) lymph plexus drains through the diaphragm to anterior mediastinal nodes, and on its under surface to nodes in the porta hepatis. The deep plexus drains to the posterior mediastinal and porta hepatis nodes.

c **F**— Parasympathetic fibres from both vagi supply the liver via the anterior gastric nerve; sympathetic fibres supply it from the coeliac plexus along the hepatic arteries.

d **T**— The bare area of the posterior surface is closely related to the diaphragm, inferior vena cava and right suprarenal gland.

e **T**— Via the hepatic artery, this ascends in the lesser omentum to divide at the porta hepatis into right and left branches.

a **T**— At the duodenal papilla on the medial wall of the descending part of the duodenum.

b **T**— Behind the superior part of the duodenum it lies anterior to the portal vein.

c **T**— Behind the head of the pancreas it lies anterior to the inferior vena cava.

d **F**— Both these ducts open into the ampulla, whose entry into the duodenum is guarded by a sphincter of smooth muscle which may also guard the duodenal opening.

e **F**— These join in the porta to form the common hepatic duct and this is joined by the cystic duct to form the bile duct.

a **F**— Its fundus is in contact with the anterior abdominal wall deep to the tip of the ninth right costal cartilage.

b **T**— Its fundus and body lie immediately anterior to the descending and superior parts of the duodenum.

c **T**— The cystic artery.

d **F**— Columnar epithelium lines the whole biliary tract. In the gall bladder are numerous mucus-secreting goblet cells.

e **F**— It lies on the inferior surface of the liver with only its fundus and the inferior surface of the body covered with peritoneum.

94 The spleen:
a lies deep to the left 9th, 10th and 11th ribs. ( )
b is separated by the diaphragm from the chest wall. ( )
c is closely related to the stomach. ( )
d is separated by the stomach from the tail of the pancreas. ( )
e is closely related to the left kidney. ( )

95 The pancreas:
a is completely invested in peritoneum. ( )
b usually has two major ducts. ( )
c is related to both the greater sac of peritoneum and the omental bursa. ( )
d lies anterior to the right and left renal veins. ( )
e is closely related to the bile duct. ( )

96 The kidneys:
a lie with their hila at the level of the 4th lumbar vertebra. ( )
b lie in a fascial sheath with their related suprarenal gland. ( )
c are related posteriorly to the lower ribs. ( )
d possess a hilus on their medial border in which the pelvis of the ureter lies anterior to the renal artery and posterior to the renal vein. ( )
e drain lymph to para-aortic lymph glands. ( )

a **T**— It lies behind the left midaxillary line deep to these ribs
b **T** being separated by the diaphragm from them and the left pleural sac.
c **T**— Its anterior surface is directly related to the greater curvature of the stomach.
d **F**— The tail of the pancreas extends in the lienorenal ligament to the hilus of the spleen.
e **T**— The posterior surface is closely related to the left kidney and suprarenal gland.

a **F**— It is covered by peritoneum anteriorly and inferiorly (the attachment of the transverse mesocolon) across the posterior abdominal wall from the duodenum to the spleen.
b **T**— The main pancreatic duct joins the bile duct in the ampulla and opens about the middle of the medial wall of the descending duodenum. The accessory duct draining the uncinate process may open separately into the duodenum proximal to the duodenal papilla, but frequently joins the main pancreatic duct.
c **T**— The transverse mesocolon which is attached to the border between the anterior and inferior surfaces of the gland separates these two peritoneal sacs.
d **T**— Both renal veins join the inferior vena cava behind the head of the pancreas.
e **T**— The bile duct extends posteriorly and passes into the gland as it approaches the ampulla; here it usually joins the pancreatic duct.

a **F**— Their hila lie close to the transpyloric plane, at the level of the 2nd lumbar vertebra.
b **F**— They are surrounded by perirenal fat and enclosed by part of the fascia tansversalis which separates each of them from a suprarenal gland.
c **T**— The diaphragm separates them from the 11th and 12th ribs.
d **F**— At the hilus of each kidney the renal vein, artery and pelvis of the ureter lie in that order from before backward.

e **T**— These lie around the origin of the renal arteries.

97   The left kidney:
a   is separated from the psoas major muscle by
the quadratus lumborum muscle.   (   )
b   is crossed posteriorly by the body of the pancreas. (   )

c   has cubial epithelium with a brush border lining
the proximal convoluted tubule.   (   )
d   develops from the pronephros.   (   )

e   is closely related to the splenic vessels.   (   )

98   The ureters:
a   have an abdominal course which is different in
each sex.   (   )

b   lie anterior to branches of the lumbar plexus and
posterior to the anterior branches of the aorta.   (   )

c   have a pelvic course which is different in each sex. (   )
d   turn medially over levator ani at the level of the
ischial spine.   (   )

e   gain a sensory nerve supply from the autonomic
nervous system.   (   )

99   The suprarenal gland:
a   on the right side lies on the right crus of the
diaphragm.   (   )
b   on the left side lies on the left crus of the diaphragm. (   )
c   on each side is related to the inferior vena cava.   (   )

d   receives its nerve supply from branches of the
thoracic sympathetic trunk.   (   )
e   lies alongside the coeliac axis.   (   )

a **F**— The kidney lies anterior to both muscles and to the transversus abdominis muscle.

b **F**— The body of the pancreas passes in front of the hilus and middle third of the kidney. The tail of the pancreas lies in the lienorenal ligament.

c **T**— This part of the nephron (functional unit of the kidney) is responsible for water reabsorption.

d **F**— The secreting part of the kidney develops from the metanephros. The collecting system (beyond the distal convoluted tubule) develops from the ureteric bud of the mesonephric duct.

e **T**— These pass anteriorly to the hilus and middle part of the kidney.

a **F**— The abdominal course of each ureter is similar in male and female; their courses in the pelvis are different in the two sexes.

b **T**— Both ureters descend on psoas, crossing over the genitofemoral nerve and being crossed over by the gonadal vessels. On the right side, the ureter is also crossed over by the duodenum and the right colic and ileocolic vessels: on the left side by the left colic vessels and the sigmoid colon.

c **T**— In both sexes the ureter crosses the bifurcation of the
d **T** common iliac vessels in front of the sacro-iliac joint and descends to the ischial spine before turning medially. In the male the ductus deferens crosses over it at this point, whereas in the female it runs medially under the root of the broad ligament being crossed over by the uterine artery and lying close to the lateral vaginal fornix, before entering the bladder.

e **T**— These nerve fibres originate in the upper lumbar and sacral segments of the cord.

a **T**— The right gland is pyramidal, the left crescentic, and both
b **T** have a rich blood supply from neighbouring arteries.

c **F**— The inferior vena cava lies anterior to the right suprarenal. The two glands are separated by the coeliac plexus with which they are intimately connected, and by the aorta.

d **T**— Via the splanchnic nerves. Preganglionic fibres end in the medulla of the gland.

e **T**— The two glands are separated by the coeliac plexus lying in front of the aorta.

100   The psoas major muscle:
a   is attached to the middle of the sides of the
lumbar vertebral bodies.   (   )

b   is attached to the lesser trochanter of the femur.   (   )

c   receives its nerve supply from all the lumbar nerves. (   )
d   both flexes the hip joint and the trunk.   (   )

e   gains attachment to the femur by passing below
the pubic rami.   (   )

101   The thoracolumbar fascia:
a   lies posterior to the muscles of the posterior
abdominal wall.   (   )
b   gives attachment to both the internal oblique
and transversus abdominis muscles.   (   )

c   is attached medially to the spinous processes
of the lumbar and sacral vertebrae.   (   )
d   is attached medially to the lumbar transverse
processes.   (   )

e   connects the iliac crest to the 12th rib.   (   )

102   The lumbar part of the lumbosacral plexus:
a   lies in the substance of psoas major.   (   )
b   is formed by the dorsal rami of all the lumbar nerves.(   )

c   has no cutaneous branches.   (   )

d   contributes to the sacral part of the lumbosacral
plexus.   (   )
e   contributes nerve fibres to the sciatic nerve.   (   )

a F— It is attached to fibrous arches which cross the concave sides of the lumbar vertebrae, to the edges of the bodies of the lumbar vertebrae and the discs between, and to the lumbar transverse processes.

b T— As it approaches the femur, it is joined by the iliacus muscle on its lateral side.

c F— It is supplied by branches of the 1st and 2nd lumbar nerves.

d T— Contraction will produce flexion and medial rotation at the hip joint, or flexion of the lumbar region of the trunk on the femur.

e F— It gains the thigh by passing under the inguinal ligament, above the superior pubic ramus.

a F— It consists of three fascial layers which enclose the posterior abdominal wall muscles. The layers fuse at the

b T   lateral limit of the muscles and become continuous with the aponeuroses of the internal oblique and transversus abdominis muscles.

c T— The strong posterior layer covers erector spinae and is attached to the lumbar and sacral spinous processes; the

d T   middle layer is attached medially to the ends of the lumbar transverse processes; the thin anterior layer covers quadratus lumborum and is attached to the front of the base of the lumbar transverse processes.

e T— Superiorly it is thickened to form the lateral cruciate ligament.

a T

b F— It is usually formed by the ventral rami of the first four lumbar nerves.

c F— The iliohypogastric and ilioinguinal nerves arise from it and supply the skin of the anterior abdominal wall and the external genitalia; the genitofemoral nerve supplies skin over the genitalia and the femoral triangle; the lateral femoral cutaneous nerve supplies skin over the lateral aspect of the thigh. Peritoneum is also supplied.

d T— By the lumbosacral trunk which is formed by the 4th and 5th lumbar nerves.

e T— Via the lumbosacral trunk (L4, L5) which descends over the sacrum to join the lumbosacral plexus.

103   The abdominal aorta:
a   ends anterior to the body of the 4th lumbar
    vertebra.   (   )
b   has the cisterna chyli lying on its left side.   (   )

c   has the inferior vena cava lying on its right side.   (   )

d   is related anteriorly to the right renal vein.   (   )
e   lies in close relationship with the lumbar vertebrae.   (   )

104   The renal arteries:
a   arise from the aorta at the level of the 2nd
    lumbar vertebra.   (   )
b   are both related posteriorly to the crus of the
    diaphragm of the same side.   (   )

c   supply branches to the corresponding suprarenal
    gland and ureter.   (   )
d   give testicular (or ovarian) branches.   (   )

e   are of unequal length; the left artery is longer than
    the right.   (   )

105   The inferior vena cava:
a   is formed on the front of the 3rd lumbar vertebra
    by the union of the two common iliac veins.   (   )
b   leaves the abdomen via the caval opening of the
    diaphragm at the level of the 8th thoracic vertebra.   (   )
c   receives tributaries from both gonadal veins.   (   )

d   receives several hepatic veins.   (   )

e   lies to the left of the aorta.   (   )

a T— Here it bifurcates into the two common iliac arteries.

b F— The cisterna chyli lies between the right side of the aorta and the right crus of the diaphragm.

c T— The cisterna chyli and the right crus lie between the aorta and the inferior vena cava which also lies further to the right.

d F— The left renal vein crosses it anteriorly.

e T— It lies directly anterior to the bodies of the upper four lumbar vertebrae.

a T— Arising at this level, the right renal artery crosses the right crus of the diaphragm lying behind the head of the

b T pancreas and the inferior vena cava. The shorter left renal artery crosses the left crus lying behind the body of the pancreas.

c T— Each renal artery gives branches to the suprarenal gland and the upper part of the ureter.

d F— The gonadal vessels arise directly from the aorta at the level of the 3rd lumbar vertebra and course down the posterior abdominal wall crossing over the ureter, the genitofemoral nerve and the psoas muscle.

e F— The aorta lies to the left of the midline, hence the left renal artery is the shorter.

a F— It is formed in front of the 5th lumbar vertebra.

b T— The caval opening lies in the central tendon of the diaphragm to the right of the midline.

c F— The left gonadal vein drains into the left renal vein, the right is a tributary of the inferior vena cava.

d T— The hepatic veins usually comprise two or three large vessels and a variable number of smaller vessels. They enter the part of the vena cava which is usually embedded in the liver.

e F— The left ureter lies along its left side.

V   Pelvis and Perineum

106 **The ilium of the hip bone:**
  a   forms two-fifths of the acetabulum.   (   )

  b   has a subcutaneous upper border.   (   )

  c   gives attachment to the rectus femoris muscle.   (   )

  d   gives attachment to the adductor magnus muscle.   (   )
  e   gives attachment to the inguinal ligament.   (   )

107 **The sacrum:**
  a   is formed of four fused sacral vertebrae.   (   )
  b   has foramina communicating with the central
      sacral canal.   (   )

  c   gives attachment to piriformis on the lateral
      part of its dorsal surface.   (   )
  d   gives attachment to the erector spinae muscles
      on the medial part of its dorsal surface.   (   )
  e   is closely related to the rectum.   (   )

108 **The sacro-iliac joint:**
  a   is a fibrous joint in a young person.   (   )

  b   owes its stability to the neighbouring muscles.   (   )

  c   allows only slight rotation and gliding movements
      to occur.   (   )

  d   lies behind the bifurcation of the common iliac
      vessels and the ureter.   (   )

  e   lies anterior to the sciatic nerve.   (   )

a **T**— It contributes the upper two-fifths of this articular surface. The ischium contributes the posterior two-fifths and the pubis the remainder.

b. **T**— The iliac crest extends from the anterior to the posterior superior iliac spine and is subcutaneous throughout most of its length. Its uppermost part lies at the level of the body and spine of the 3rd lumbar vertebra. The line joining the highest points marks the supracristal plane and is a surface marking for a lumbar puncture.

c **T**— This strong flexor of the thigh at the hip joint is attached to the anterior inferior iliac spine and the adjacent ilium.

d **F**— This muscle is attached along the ischiopubic ramus.

e **T**— The lateral end of the inguinal ligament is attached to the anterior border of the ilium at the anterior superior iliac spine.

a **F**— Five vertebrae usually fuse and form it.

b **T**— Paired pelvic and dorsal foramina communicate by corresponding intervertebral foramina with the central sacral canal and convey ventral and dorsal rami of the sacral nerves.

c **F**— Piriformis is attached to the pelvic surface of the lateral mass of the sacrum.

d **T**— The erector spinae arises in part from this surface which also gives attachment to the thoracolumbar fascia.

e **T**— The lower part of its anterior (pelvic) surface lies in contact with the rectum.

a **F**— It is a synovial joint of the plane variety between the sacrum and ilium. In adults the joint cavity may be partly obliterated by fibrous adhesions.

b **F**— Stability is maintained almost entirely by very strong ligaments — i.e. the interosseous, dorsal and ventral sacro-iliac, the sacrotuberous and the sacrospinous ligaments.

c **T**— The weight of the trunk tends to rotate the promontory of the sacrum forwards, this being prevented by the sacrotuberous and sacrospinous ligaments. Such gliding movement as occurs is restricted by the sacro-iliac ligaments.

d **T**— The lumbosacral trunk, obturator nerve and psoas muscle are also anterior to the joint, separating the joint from the iliac vessels.

e **F**— Posteriorly it is covered only by the erector spinae and gluteus maximus muscles.

109   **The symphysis pubis:**
   a   is a secondary cartilaginous joint.   (   )

   b   has its surfaces covered with fibrocartilage.   (   )
   c   allows little or no movement.   (   )
   d   gains most of its stability from accessory ligaments.   (   )
   e   is united by a fibrocartilaginous disc.   (   )

110   **The lesser pelvis:**
   a   in the female, has a relatively longer anteroposterior
        diameter at the pelvic inlet.   (   )

   b   has an outlet bounded by the ischiopubic rami
        and the sacrotuberous ligaments.   (   )
   c   has a cavity whose anterior wall is much shorter
        than the posterior.   (   )
   d   has a smaller subpubic angle in the female than
        in the male.   (   )
   e   in the female is generally circular in cross section.   (   )

111   **The levator ani muscle:**
   a   gains attachment from the fascia covering obturator
        internus.   (   ).
   b   gains attachment to both the perineal body and the
        anococcygeal body.   (   )
   c   reinforces both the rectal and urethral sphincters.   (   )

   d   is supplied largely by sympathetic and
        parasympathetic nerves.   (   )
   e   forms all of the pelvic floor.   (   )

a **T**— As are many other midline joints, such as the manubriosternal and all the intervertebral discs.

b **F**— Hyaline cartilage covers the joint surfaces.

c **T**— Except in the later stages of pregnancy.

d **F**— The joint is strengthened on all surfaces by interpubic

e **T** ligaments and by its attachments to the intra-articular disc. It possesses no accessory ligaments.

a **F**— During parturition the fetal head enters the lesser pelvis in the transverse diameter and emerges through the outlet in the anteroposterior diameter. The head of a postmature fetus may be too large and a Caesarian section may be necessary.

b **T**— The outlet is diamond-shaped and, in the female, the anteroposterior diameter is greater than the transverse.

c **T**— In both sexes the cavity is a short curved cavity whose posterior wall is about three times longer than the anterior.

d **F**— The angle is more than 90° in the female, and less in the male.

e **F**— The maximum diameter of the inlet is transverse and of the outlet anteroposterior. Hence, in normal labour the head undergoes partial rotation during descent.

a **T**— Laterally it is attached to the back of the body of the pubis, the fascia covering obturator internus and the ischial spine.

b **T**— Its fibres descend to the midline to meet the opposite muscle in a midline raphe. The anterior fibres pass around

c **T** the urethra and prostate (or the urethra and vagina) to the fibrous perineal body; the middle fibres pass medially around the rectum to the anococcygeal body; and the posterior fibres pass to the midline raphe and the coccyx. It provides muscular support for the pelvic viscera and reinforces the rectal and urethral sphincters.

d **F**— It is supplied by branches of the 3rd and 4th sacral nerves and the pudendal nerve and is under voluntary control.

e **F**— The two coccygei muscles contribute to the posterior part of the pelvic floor.

true or false

112   The pelvic floor:
a   is formed by levator ani and coccygeus.   (   )

b   separates the perineum from the ischiorectal fossae.   (   )

c   is covered superiorly by fascia.   (   )
d   has the pelvic vessels and nerves on its
      undersurface.   (   )

e   is gutter shaped.   (   )

113   The rectum:
a   begins in front of the 1st sacral vertebra.   (   )
b   has no mesentery.   (   )

c   forms the posterior wall of a peritoneal pouch.   (   )
d   in the male is related anteriorly to the seminal
      vesicles and prostate.   (   )

e   is related anteriorly to the cervix.   (   )

114   The rectum:
a   is related posteriorly to the 3rd, 4th and 5th
      sacral nerves.   (   )
b   has a lining of stratified squamous epithelium.   (   )

c   has a venous drainage into the superior
      mesenteric vein.   (   )

d   sends lymph vessels to the superficial inguinal
      nodes.   (   )

e   is a straight structure.   (   )

a **T**— It is formed by the two levator ani muscles anteriorly and the two coccygei posteriorly.

b **F**— It is a fibromuscular diaphragm separating the pelvic cavity above from the perineum and ischiorectal fossae below.

c **T**— The tough pelvic fascia covers it superiorly.

d **F**— Both the vessels and nerves lie on the superior surface of the pelvic floor. The pudendal vessels and nerves lie below.

e **T**— This gutter-like arrangement rotates the fetal head as it descends through the pelvis.

a **F**— It begins in front of the 3rd sacral vertebra.

b **T**— Its upper third is covered by peritoneum on its front and sides, its middle third on its front only, and its lower third lies embedded in the pelvic fascia.

c **T**— Its upper two-thirds form the rectovesical pouch in the

d **T** male, and the rectouterine pouch in the female. In its lower part its anterior relations may be palpated by digital examination of the rectum. These are the vagina and cervix in the female, and the prostate, seminal vesicles and ducti deferentia in the male.

e **T**— On digital examination of the female, the cervix is palpable through the rectal wall.

a **T**— Also to the sympathetic plexus, the sacrum and the piriformis muscle.

b **F**— The lining is of columnar epithelium, containing numerous mucous glands and aggregations of lymphoid tissue.

c **F**— The superior rectal vein is a tributary of the inferior mesenteric vein. There are also important anastomoses with the inferior rectal branch of the internal pudendal vein.

d **F**— These nodes drain the lower anal canal. The rectal drainage passes along the superior rectal vessels to the pre-aortic nodes and laterally to the internal iliac nodes.

e **F**— It curves anteriorly as it descends and usually loops toward the left side of the pelvis.

115   The anal canal:
a   possesses an internal sphincter of voluntary muscle. (   )
b   possesses an external sphincter supplied by
parasympathetic nerves.   (   )

c   is adjacent to the ischiorectal fossa.   (   )

d   has a lymph drainage to both the nodes around
the common iliac vein and to the superficial
inguinal nodes.   (   )

e   is lined by both columnar and squamous epithelium. (   )

116   The urinary bladder:
a   has no peritoneal covering.   (   )

b   is lined with cubical epithelium.   (   )
c   is attached to the umbilicus.   (   )

d   is closely related to the pubic bones.   (   )

e   has a lymphatic drainage to the inguinal nodes.   (   )

117   The urinary bladder:
a   has a motor nerve supply from both the
sympathetic and parasympathetic systems.   (   )
b   has a sensory supply from both sympathetic and
parasympathetic systems.   (   )
c   has a venous drainage to the inferior mesenteric
vein.   (   )
d   is largely supported by the pelvic fascia.   (   )

e   lies in close contact with the vagina.   (   )

a **F**— The internal sphincter is an involuntary muscle and a
b **F**   continuation of the rectum's circular muscle coat. The
external sphincter encircles the lower two-thirds of the anal
canal and is arranged into deep, superficial and
subcutaneous parts. It is voluntary muscle supplied by the
inferior rectal nerves and is reinforced by the levator ani
muscle.

c **T**— It is separated from it by the levator ani and the external
sphincter muscles.

d **T**— The upper two-thirds of the anal canal drain to the nodes
around the common iliac vein and the pre-aortic nodes.
The lower anal canal drains to the superficial inguinal
nodes.

e **T**— The lower one-third is lined with squamous epithelium. It
joins that part lined with columnar epithelium at the
dentate line.

a **F**— Its superior surface in both sexes is covered by peritoneum
and the upper part of the posterior surface in the male.

b **F**— The mucosa is lined with transitional epithelium.

c **T**— The median umbilical ligament, a remnant of the urachus,
ascends to the umbilicus.

d **T**— The anterolateral surfaces, though separated slightly from
the pubic bones by a fat-filled retropubic space, lie close
enough for bladder injuries to complicate pubic fractures.

e **F**— It drains to external and internal iliac nodes.

a **T**— Both sympathetic and parasympathetic fibres supply the
bladder; the sympathetic is motor to the vesical sphincter,
b **T**   the parasympathetic to the bladder wall. Sensory fibres are
found in both supplies.

c **F**— It drains via the vesical venous plexus to the internal iliac
veins.

d **T**— Pelvic fascia surrounds the bladder and the fascial
thickenings around its neck attach it to the pubis
(pubovesical and puboprostatic ligaments) and to the
pelvic wall (lateral ligaments of the bladder).

e **T**— It lies anterior to the vagina.

118   The uterus:
  a   is an anterior relation of the anal canal.   (   )
  b   is supported by the parametrium.   (   )

  c   is crossed laterally above its middle by the ureter.   (   )
  d   sends its lymph vessels to the common iliac nodes.   (   )

  e   lies in the line of the vagina.   (   )

119   The broad ligament of the uterus:
  a   extends from the uterus to the lateral surface of the
       bladder.   (   )
  b   contains the uterine tube.   (   )

  c   contains the suspensory ligament of the ovary.   (   )

  d   contains the round ligament of the uterus.   (   )

  e   contains parametrium.   (   )

120   The uterine tubes:
  a   lie in the base of the uterine broad ligament.   (   )
  b   in the adult are about 4 cm long.   (   )
  c   are lined by ciliated epithelium.   (   )
  d   extend to the medial surface of the ovary.   (   )

  e   are, when healthy, always patent.   (   )

a **F**— The anal canal lies posterior to the vagina.
b **T**— The parametrium consists of strong bands of pelvic fascia radiating from the cervix to the pelvic walls. The lateral (cardinal) ligaments are the largest.
c **F**— The ureter is a lateral relation of the lateral vaginal fornix.
d **T**— Some vessels also pass along the round ligament to the superficial inguinal nodes and some others may pass with the ovarian vessels to the para-aortic nodes.
e **F**— The uterus lies normally at right angles to the vagina.

a **F**— It is a double fold of peritoneum extending from the lateral pelvic wall to the lateral margin of the uterus.
b **T**— In the medial two-thirds of its free upper border lies the uterine tube.
c **T**— The suspensory ligament of the ovary lies in the lateral one-third of this border and contains the ovarian vessels.
d **T**— The round ligament of the uterus extends from the upper lateral angle of the uterus through the broad ligament to the deep inguinal ring, then through the inguinal canal and ends in the labium majus. It is continuous with the ovarian ligament and is a remnant of the gubernaculum of the ovary.
e **T**— This is thickened fibrous tissue which surrounds the supravaginal cervix in the base of the broad ligament.

a **F**— The tubes lie in the upper borders of the broad ligament.
b **F** In the adult they are usually about 10 cm long.
c **T**— The ciliated epithelium contains many mucous cells.
d **F**— Each tube ends laterally in the fimbria which curl around and overlap the lateral surface of the ovary.
e **T**— Recurrent infection may, however, cause narrowing or closure to occur.

121   The ovary:
  a   lies on the anterior surface of the broad ligament.   (   )

  b   is related on its lateral surface to the uterine tube.   (   )

  c   lies on the lateral pelvic wall.   (   )
  d   receives a blood supply from branches of the
      uterine artery.   (   )
  e   has lymph vessels passing to internal iliac nodes.   (   )

122   The vagina:
  a   usually lies at an axis of 45° with the uterus.   (   )
  b   is related laterally to the ureter.   (   )

  c   has a lymph drainage both to iliac and superficial
      inguinal nodes.   (   )
  d   is lined with epithelium rich in mucous glands.   (   )

  e   is covered in its upper posterior part with
      peritoneum.   (   )

123   The prostate:
  a   is traversed by two ejaculatory ducts.   (   )
  b   possesses lateral and median lobes.   (   )

  c   is surrounded by a prostatic sheath and venous
      plexus.   (   )
  d   drains via its venous plexus to the internal vertebral
      venous plexus.   (   )
  e   is separated from the rectum by rectovesical fascia.   (   )

a F— It lies on the back of the broad ligament attached by a double fold of peritoneum, the mesovarium.

b T— Laterally the ovary is related to the fimbriated end of the uterine tube, and is attached to one of the fimbriae.

c T— Related to the internal iliac artery and the ureter.

d T— These supplement ovarian arteries arising from the aorta just below the renal arteries.

e F— The lymph drainage is to para-aortic nodes at the level of the renal vessels. The lymph vessels pass with the ovarian vessels.

a F— It usually lies at an angle of 90° with the uterus.

b T— Laterally it is related to the base of the broad ligament containing the ureter and uterine vessels.

c T— Its upper two-thirds drain to internal and external iliac nodes, its lower third to superficial inguinal nodes.

d F— Its squamous epithelial lining containing no glands. The greater vestibular glands lie laterally.

e T— This is the uterorectal pouch (Pouch of Douglas) separating the vagina from the rectum.

a T— These two ducts and the urethra traverse the gland and

b T with fibrous septa divide it into a median lobe lying between the urethra and ejaculatory ducts, and two lateral lobes below and lateral to the median lobe.

c T— The prostatic sheath is formed of pelvic fascia. The surrounding venous plexus drains to the internal iliac veins

d T and the internal vertebral plexus through the pelvic sacral foramina.

e T— This strong sheet of fascia covers the seminal vesicles and the front of the rectum.

124 The ductus (vas) deferens:
a is a continuation of the canal of the epididymis. (   )
b joins inferiorly with the head of the epididymis. (   )
c ends by opening into the prostatic urethra. (   )

d lies medial to the seminal vesicle. (   )

e possesses a sacculated diverticulum. (   )

125 The perineum:
a lies below the pelvic diaphragm. (   )

b is bounded anteriorly by the inguinal ligaments. (   )
c is bounded posterolaterally by the sacrotuberous
ligaments. (   )
d is bounded laterally by the ischial spines. (   )
e contains anal and perineal triangles. (   )

126 The ischiorectal fossa:
a is bounded superiorly by the levator ani muscle. (   )
b is bounded laterally by the inferior pubic ramus. (   )
c does not communicate with its fellow of the
opposite side. (   )

d is related medially to the anal canal. (   )
e contains the seminal vesicles. (   )

a **T**— It is a narrow muscular tube extending from the tail of the
b **F** epididymis and, joining with the duct of the seminal
c **F** vesicle, forms the 2 cm long ejaculatory duct which opens
into the prostatic urethra.
d **T**— In its terminal part it descends posterior to the bladder and
medial to the seminal vesicle.
e **T**— This is the seminal vesicle and it lies behind the base of
the bladder.

a **T**— It is the diamond-shaped space between the pubic
symphysis and the coccyx.
b **F**— It is bounded anteriorly by the ischiopubic rami,
c **T** posterolaterally by the sacrotuberous ligaments and
laterally by the ischial tuberosities.
d **F**
e **F**— A line joining the ischial tuberosities divides the perineum
into an anterior urogenital and a posterior anal triangle.

a **T**— It is a wedge-shaped space, bounded superomedially by
b **F** levator ani, laterally by the fascia on obturator internus
c **F** and inferiorly by perineal skin. The two fossae
communicate with each other around the anal canal and
are separated by the anococcygeal body, the anal canal
and the perineal body.
d **T**
e **F**— The vesicles lie above the levator ani and so are within the
pelvis. The fat-filled fossa extends forwards towards the
pubis and backwards towards the sacrum. The pudendal
canal is on the lateral wall.

127   The urogenital diaphragm:
a   is attached to the ischiopubic rami.   (   )
b   is attached to the anococcygeal body.   (   )

c   in the female, is pierced by the vagina as well
     as the urethra.   (   )

d   has, between its two layers, the vesical sphincter.   (   )

e   gives attachment to perineal muscles.   (   )

128   The superficial perineal pouch:
a   is limited inferiorly by the urogenital diaphragm.   (   )

b   is continuous with the spaces in the scrotum
     occupied by the testes.   (   )

c   has a membranous covering which provides a
     fascial sheath around the penis.   (   )
d   contains the penis, testes and spermatic cords.   (   )
e   is traversed by the urethra in the male and the
     urethra and vagina in the female.   (   )

129   The penis:
a   comprises two cylinders of erectile tissue.   (   )
b   contains a ventral corpus spongiosum which
     expands anteriorly to form the glans penis.   (   )
c   contains corpora cavernosa which expand
     posteriorly to form the bulb of the penis.   (   )

d   has a lymph drainage to the internal iliac nodes.   (   )
e   has veins draining to the prostatic plexus.   (   )

a **T**— This double layer of fascia stretches across the pubic arch
b **F** between the ischiopubic rami. Its posterior border is
attached to the perineal body.
c **T**— In the female it is a less well-defined structure but attached
to its inferior surface are the bulb of the vestibule, the
greater vestibular glands and the small crura of the clitoris.
In the male the bulb surrounding the urethra and the large
crura of the penis are attached to its inferior surface and
the adjacent ischiopubic rami.
d **F**— The urethral sphincter occupies this position. It is
composed of voluntary muscle, supplied by the perineal
branch of the pudendal nerve.
e **T**— In the male it also gives attachment to the bulb and crura
of the penis.

a **F**— It lies between the urogenital diaphragm superiorly, and
inferiorly the membranous layer of the superficial fascia
which is continuous with that of the anterior abdominal
wall.
b **T**— The membranous layer of superficial fascia passes over the
scrotum to be attached to the posterior border of the
urogenital diaphragm.
c **T**— The pouch contains the bulb and crura of the penis (and
corresponding structures in the female) and the superficial
d **T** perineal muscles.
e **T**— In the female, the greater vestibular glands are also found
in the pouch.

a **F**— There are three longitudinal cylinders of erectile tissue.
b **T**— The unpaired ventral corpus spongiosum expands
anteriorly and forms the glans penis, and posteriorly it
c **F** forms the bulb of the penis. The two united, dorsally-
placed corpora cavernosa diverge posteriorly and form the
crura of the penis.
d **F**— It drains to the superficial inguinal group of nodes.
e **T**— Together with branches to the internal pudendal veins.

130   The male urethra:
a   receives a midline ejaculatory duct.   (   )
b   receives two prostatic ducts.   (   )

c   traverses the whole length of the corpus
    spongiosum.   (   )
d   has the sphincter urethrae muscle surrounding its
    prostatic part.   (   )

e   is narrowest in its membranous part.   (   )

131   The pudendal nerve:
a   arises from the lumbar plexus.   (   )
b   traverses the greater sciatic foramen.   (   )
c   traverses the lesser sciatic foramen.   (   )

d   supplies levator ani and perianal skin.   (   )

e   supplies sensory fibres to the penis.   (   )

132   The common iliac arteries:
a   arise in front of the promontory of the sacrum.   (   )
b   have no branches other than the terminal internal
    and external iliac arteries.   (   )
c   lie in front and to the right of the internal iliac veins. (   )
d   are closely related to the inferior vena cava.   (   )
e   are crossed at their origin by the ureters.   (   )

133   The external iliac artery:
a   ends behind the inguinal ligament at the
    midinguinal point.   (   )
b   lies on the psoas major muscle.   (   )
c   is crossed anteriorly by the ureter.   (   )

d   is crossed anteriorly by the gonadal vessels.   (   )
e   supplies blood to the anterior abdominal wall.   (   )

a **F**— The posterior wall of the prostatic urethra is marked by an
b **F** elevation, the prostatic utricle on each side of which enters
an ejaculatory duct. Into the groove on each lateral side
open the 20–30 prostatic ducts.
c **T**— The spongy urethra is some 16 cm long and it traverses
the whole length of the corpus spongiosum.
d **F**— The sphincter urethrae surrounds the narrow membranous
urethra and is formed of striated (voluntary) muscle. The
sphincter lies between the prostate and bulb, and is
supplied by the perineal branch of the pudendal nerve.
e **T**— Where it descends through the deep perineal pouch.

a **F**— It arises from the sacral plexus.
b **T**— It leaves the pelvis through the greater sciatic foramen,
c **T** crosses the ischial spine and enters the perineum through
the lesser sciatic foramen to pass forwards in the pudendal
canal.
d **T**— Together with the external anal and urethral sphincters,
perineal muscles and scrotal (labial) skin.
e **T**— Via branches of the dorsal nerve of the penis.

a **F**— They arise in front of the body of the fourth lumbar vertebra.
b **T**— They end by dividing, anterior to the sacro-iliac joints, into
these terminal branches.
c **F**— They lie anterior and to the left of the internal iliac veins. The
d **T** origin of the inferior vena cava lies behind the right artery.
e **F**— The ureters cross anteriorly the terminal bifurcation of the
common iliac arteries.

a **T**— At this point it continues into the thigh as the femoral artery.
It is palpable at this point.
b **T**— Throughout its course it lies anterior to the psoas muscle.
c **F**— It is crossed anteriorly by the testicular or ovarian vessels
and the ductus deferens. The ureter crosses the bifurcation
d **T** of the common iliac artery.
e **T**— The inferior epigastric artery arises just above the inguinal
ligament, ascends the inner aspect of the abdominal wall
medial to the deep inguinal ring, and enters the sheath of
rectus abdominis. It anastomoses with the superior epigastric
artery.

134   The cisterna chyli:
a   drains directly into the left jugular vein.   (   )
b   lies between the right crus of the diaphragm and
     the aorta.   (   )
c   receives the right and left lumbar lymph trunks.   (   )
d   receives lymph (chyle) from the abdominal
     alimentary tract.   (   )

e   receives all the lymph from the anterior abdominal
     wall.   (   )

135   The sacral part of the lumbosacral plexus:
a   is formed by the ventral rami of the 4th and 5th
     lumbar nerves and the upper four sacral nerves.   (   )
b   lies on iliacus muscle.   (   )

c   gives branches to the gluteal muscles.   (   )
d   gives branches to supply the skin of the buttock
     and the perineum.   (   )

e   supplies the coccygeal plexus.   (   )

136   The coeliac plexus:
a   is formed of two interconnecting coeliac ganglia.   (   )
b   receives branches from both vagal trunks.   (   )

c   gives branches which end in the suprarenal medulla. (   )

d   supplies branches to the alimentary tract and
     urogenital tract.   (   )

e   conveys visceral pain fibres.   (   )

a **F**— It leads directly into the thoracic duct as it passes through
b **T** the diaphragm between its right crus and the aorta.

c **T**— The lumbar lymph trunks are formed by the efferents of
d **T** the para-aortic nodes; the intestinal lymph trunk is formed
by the efferents of the pre-aortic lymph nodes. All drain
into the cisterna chyli.
e **F**— Though the lower half drains into inguinal nodes, that from
the upper part drains to axillary nodes and thence to the
thoracic duct.

a **T**

b **F**— It lies in front of the sacrum on the surface of piriformis
deep to the pelvic fascia.
c **T**— The superior and inferior gluteal nerves.
d **T**— The perforating cutaneous nerve supplies the skin of the
medial part of the buttock and the perineal branch of the
4th sacral nerve supplies the perianal skin. The sciatic and
obturator nerves also arise from the sacral plexus.
e **F**— This is formed of the 4th and 5th sacral nerves. It lies on
coccygeus and supplies the skin over the coccyx.

a **T**— Which lie on each side of the origin of the coeliac artery.
b **T**— It is a plexus of both parasympathetic and sympathetic
nerves receiving branches from the thoracic sympathetic
trunk via the greater, lesser and least splanchnic nerves
and parasympathetic branches from the anterior and
posterior vagal trunks.
c **T**— Presynaptic fibres from the sympathetic trunks pass
through the plexus and supply the suprarenal medulla
directly.
d **T**— Postsynaptic fibres pass with the aorta and its branches
and supply the upper part of the alimentary tract, the
kidneys and gonads.
e **T**— Afferent pain fibres from the viscera are conveyed by
parasympathetic fibres through this plexus.

VI The Upper Limb

137 The clavicle:
a has no medullary cavity.　　　　　　　　　　　　( )

b is convex anteriorly in the medial two-thirds.　( )
c laterally gives attachment to trapezius.　　　　( )

d stabilises the shoulder joint.　　　　　　　　　( )

e articulates laterally with the coracoid process of the
   scapula.　　　　　　　　　　　　　　　　　( )

138 The scapula has a:
a palpable inferior angle which overlies the seventh
   rib.　　　　　　　　　　　　　　　　　　　( )

b lateral border giving rise to the serratus anterior
   muscle.　　　　　　　　　　　　　　　　　( )
c costal surface divided by a projecting spine into
   supraspinous and infraspinous fossae.　　　　( )
d coracoid process giving attachment to the biceps
   muscle.　　　　　　　　　　　　　　　　　( )

e glenoid cavity, below which the long head of the
   triceps muscle is attached.　　　　　　　　　( )

139 In the humerus the:
a subscapularis muscle is attached to the greater
   tuberosity.　　　　　　　　　　　　　　　　( )
b greater tuberosity is separated from the lesser
   tuberosity by the intertubercular groove.　　　( )
c upper end has a V-shaped tuberosity for the
   attachment of the deltoid muscle.　　　　　　( )
d olecranon fossa gives attachment to the medial
   head of the triceps muscle.　　　　　　　　　( )

e axillary nerve lies medial to the anatomical
   neck.　　　　　　　　　　　　　　　　　　( )

a T— Though a long bone, it is also atypical in its largely membranous development.

b T— The lateral third is concave anteriorly.

c T— Trapezius gains attachment to the posterior aspect of its lateral third.

d F— Its important functions are those of support to the upper limb and as an 'outrigger' which thrusts the scapula away from the chest wall, thus increasing the range of movement at the shoulder joint.

e F— The flattened lateral end articulates with the medial side of the acromion. Strong ligaments joining the clavicle to the coracoid process act as a fulcrum for movement.

a T— The scapula covers the posterolateral aspect of the chest wall over the 2nd to the 7th ribs and its subcutaneous inferior angle is an important surface landmark.

b F— The muscle arises from the dorsal surface of the medial border.

c F— The costal surface is concave and has no spine. The dorsal surface is divided in this way by a subcutaneous spine.

d T— Biceps is attached to the scapula by two heads; the short head to the coracoid process and the long head to a tubercle above the glenoid cavity.

e T— The other two heads are attached to the humerus, bordering the radial groove.

a F— The muscle is attached to the lesser tuberosity.

b T— The groove houses the long tendon of the biceps.

c F— The deltoid is attached halfway down the lateral surface of the body of the humerus.

d F— The fossa is for the olecranon process of the ulnar, the muscle gains attachment to the posterior aspect of the humerus below the radial groove.

e F— The nerve lies medial to the surgical neck and is susceptible to injury in fractures of the surgical neck or dislocation of the shoulder joint.

140   **The sternoclavicular joint:**

a   is a synovial joint.   ( )
b   is of the ellipsoid variety.   ( )

c   has joint surfaces lined by fibrocartilage.   ( )
d   owes most of its stability to its capsular ligaments.   ( )

e   lies anterior to the aortic arch.   ( )

141   **The acromioclavicular joint:**

a   is not a synovial joint.   ( )
b   typically contains a disc of hyaline cartilage.   ( )
c   gains its stability from its capsular ligament.   ( )
d   possesses no accessory ligaments.   ( )

e   lies in close proximity to the brachial plexus.   ( )

142   **The shoulder joint:**

a   has a scapular articular surface less than one-third
    that of the humeral head.   ( )

b   is surrounded by a tight capsular ligament.   ( )

c   usually communicates superiorly with the
    subacromial bursa.   ( )
d   depends for most of its stability on the capsular
    and accessory ligaments.   ( )

e   is closely related inferiorly to the axillary nerve.   ( )

a **T**— It has a small range of movement.
b **F**— It is a ball and socket joint capable of elevation, depression, forward and backward movement in a horizontal plane, circumduction and axial rotation.
c **T**— Its joint surfaces are lined by fibrocartilage and a
d **F** fibrocartilaginous disc completely divides the joint into medial and lateral compartments. Stability of the joint is maintained largely by the intra-articular disc and accessory joint ligaments, particularly the costoclavicular.
e **F**— Its immediate posterior relation is the origin of the brachiocephalic vein.

a **F**— It is a synovial joint of the plane variety.
b **F**— A disc is sometimes found but is rarely complete.
c **F**— The capsule is relatively weak and the joint owes its
d **F** stability to its two accessory ligaments, particularly the strong coracoclavicular ligament.
e **F**— The joint lies subcutaneously and overlies the supraspinatus muscle.

a **T**— Even though the scapular articular surface is extended by the ring of fibrocartilage, the glenoidal labrum, around its margin.
b **F**— The capsule is lax, particularly inferiorly, and allows for the wide range of movement at this joint.
c **F**— The subscapular bursa communicates with the joint.

d **F**— The lax capsule is of little support and the shallow glenoid cavity affords almost none. The short articular (cuff) muscles, subscapularis, supraspinatus, infraspinatus and teres minor by their close proximity are the major stabilising factors.
e **T**— Which is thus easily damaged in downward dislocation at the joint.

143 The pectoralis major muscle:

a   has a clavicular attachment to the middle third
    of the anterior surface of the clavicle.   (   )

b   has a costal attachment to the 3rd, 4th, and
    5th ribs, near the costochondral junctions.   (   )

c   has an attachment to the upper part of the external
    oblique aponeurosis.   (   )

d   is attached to the lateral lip of the lower part
    of the intertubercular groove.   (   )

e   receives its nerve supply from the lateral and
    posterior cords of the brachial plexus.   (   )

144 The serratus anterior muscle:

a   gains attachment to all of the ribs.   (   )

b   gains attachment to the medial border of the
    scapula.   (   )

c   is attached by a group of accessory fibres to the
    medial bicipital groove.   (   )

d   is an accessory muscle of respiration.   (   )

e   is supplied by the thoracodorsal branch of the
    posterior cord of the brachial plexus.   (   )

145 Trapezius is attached to the:

a   occipital bone.   (   )
b   clavicle.   (   )
c   thoracic vertebra.   (   )
d   iliac crest.   (   )
e   acromion.   (   )

a **F**— The clavicular attachment is to the medial third of the anterior surface.

b **F**— This is the costal attachment of pectoralis minor.

c **T**— The sternocostal head is also attached to the anterior surface of the sternum and the upper six costal cartilages.

d **T**— The clavicular head lies anterior to the sternocostal head at this attachment.

e **F**— The lateral and medial pectoral nerves are branches of the lateral and medial cords of the plexus.

a **F**— It arises from near the angles of the upper eight ribs and, passing forwards over the medial wall of the axilla, is attached to the medial border and inferior angle of the

b **T** scapula.

c **T**

d **T**— When the scapula is fixed, contraction will lift the upper ribs upwards and downwards.

e **F**— It is supplied by the long thoracic nerve which arises from the ventral rami of the 5th, 6th and 7th cervical nerves. The thoracodorsal nerve supplies the latissimus dorsi muscle.

a **T**— Medially it is attached to the occipital bone, the

b **T** ligamentum nuchae and the thoracic spines, and laterally

c **T** to the clavicle, acromion and spine of the scapula.

d **F**

e **T**

146   The latissimus dorsi muscle:
a   is attached to the lower six thoracic vertebrae.   (   )
b   is attached to the lumbar and sacral vertebral spines. (   )
c   has no attachment to the chest wall.   (   )

d   is attached to the inferior angle of the scapula.   (   )
e   is a powerful flexor of the humerus at the shoulder
joint.   (   )

147   The deltoid muscle:
a   is a unipennate muscle.   (   )

b   overlies the subacromial bursa.   (   )
c   is proximally attached to the clavicle, acromion
and scapular spine.   (   )

d   is distally attached to anterior upper third of the
humerus.   (   )
e   is supplied by the radial nerve.   (   )

148   The short articular (cuff) muscles of the shoulder joint:
a   comprise subscapularis, supraspinatus,
infraspinatus and teres major.   (   )

b   provide the greatest stabilising forces at the
shoulder joint.   (   )
c   provide maximal support to the inferior aspect
of the shoulder joint.   (   )
d   are all attached to the greater tuberosity of
the humerus.   (   )
e   are all supplied by branches of the posterior cord
of the brachial plexus.   (   )

a T— It is attached to the spines and supraspinous ligaments of
b T   these vertebrae and also by the thoracolumbar fascia to
c F   the lumbar and sacral spines. It is also attached to the
         lowest four ribs where it interdigitates with external
         oblique.
d T— On the dorsal aspect.
e F— It is a powerful extensor of the humerus. With the arm
         raised above the head and fixed it will pull the trunk
         upwards.

a F— It is multipennate. Strong fibrous septa intersect the
         muscle and give attachment to its fibres.
b T— Which separates it from the short articular (cuff) muscles.
c T— From this wide proximal attachment the muscle narrows
         distally to be attached to the V-shaped deltoid tuberosity
         on the lateral aspect of the humerus.
d F

e F— It is supplied by the axillary nerve. It can act as an
         abductor, flexor or extensor at the shoulder joint.

a F— The three first named muscles and teres minor lie closely
         related to the capsule of the shoulder joint (cuff muscles).
         Teres major is separated from it by a space transmitting
         the axillary nerve.
b T— Their tendons blend intimately with the capsule of the
         joint and strengthen it considerably.
c F— This is the area of least support; shoulder dislocation is
         commonest in this direction.
d F— Subscapularis is attached to the lesser tuberosity, the other
         three cuff muscles to the greater.
e F— Both supraspinatus and infraspinatus are supplied by the
         suprascapular nerve, a branch of the upper trunk of the
         brachial plexus. The other muscles are innervated from the
         posterior cord of the plexus.

149   The axilla has:

a   an apect which communicates with the posterior
triangle of neck.   (   )

b   an apex bounded in part by the medial third of the
clavicle.   (   )

c   a narrow lateral wall.   (   )

d   a posterior wall formed by serratus anterior.   (   )

e   an anterior wall containing the clavipectoral fascia. (   )

150   The axillary artery:

a   extends to the lower border of teres major.   (   )

b   lies posterior to pectoralis minor.   (   )

c   lies lateral to the medial cord of the brachial plexus. (   )

d   lies medial to the axillary vein.   (   )

e   lies lateral to the short head of biceps.   (   )

151   The scapular anastomosis:

a   provides collateral circulation between the
subclavian and brachial arteries.   (   )

b   lies closely related to the neck of the humerus. (   )

c   receives contributions from branches of the
thyrocervical trunk.   (   )

d   receives contributions from the subscapular artery. (   )

e   receives contributions from the lateral thoracic
artery.   (   )

a **T**— The apex is bounded by the superior border of the scapula, the outer border of the 1st rib and the middle
b **F**   3rd of the clavicle.

c **T**— Its lateral wall is formed by the narrow intertubercular groove of the humerus to which latissimus dorsi and teres major of the posterior axillary wall and pectoralis major of the anterior wall are attached.

d **F**— Serratus anterior, lying in the thoracic wall, forms the medial axillary boundary. The posterior wall is formed by subscapularis, latissimus dorsi and teres major.

e **T**— The fascia splits around pectoralis minor and subclavius; pectoralis major is situated anterior to these structures.

a **T**— And becomes the brachial artery.
b **T**— The artery in the axilla is surrounded by the cords and branches of the brachial plexus behind pectoralis minor.
c **T**— The cords are named because of their relationship to the artery.
d **F**— The axillary vein lies medial to the artery.
e **F**— The short head of biceps and coracobrachialis lie lateral to the artery.

a **T**— This opens up when the upper part of the axillary artery is blocked.
b **F**— It lies, as its name implies, around the scapula.
c **T**— It is formed by connections between the suprascapular artery and deep branch of the transverse cervical
d **T**   proximally and by the subscapular artery and its circumflex branch distally.
e **F**— This artery is too far anterior.

152   The brachial plexus:
a   is usually formed by the ventral rami of the lower.
      four cervical and first thoracic nerves.   (   )
b   has its roots situated posterior to the scalenus
      anterior muscle.   (   )
c   contains three trunks which lie in the neck.   (   )
d   contains three cords which lie in the neck.   (   )
e   has a posterior cord which receives contributions
      from all five roots of the plexus.   (   )

153   The brachial plexus:
a   originates from roots which emerge in front of
      scalenus anterior.   (   )

b   forms cords which are closely related to the axillary
      artery.   (   )
c   gives branches from its lateral cord to the
      extensor muscles of the upper limb.   (   )
d   supplies the latissimus dorsi muscle from its
      medial cord.   (   )
e   supplies the pectoralis major muscle.   (   )

154   The biceps muscle:
a   is attached to the scapula.   (   )

b   has an intra-articular tendon.   (   )

c   is attached to the humerus.   (   )
d   has an aponeurosis passing to the dorsal surface
      of the radius.   (   )
e   is a powerful pronator of the forearm.   (   )

a **T**— These ventral rami form the five roots of the plexus and
           unite to form three trunks in the posterior triangle of the
b **T**   neck. The upper two roots form the upper trunk, the
           middle root continues as the middle trunk and the lower
c **T**   two form the lower trunk.
d **F**— The cords are formed in the apex of the axilla behind the
e **T**   middle third of the clavicle by each trunk dividing into
           anterior and posterior divisions which then reunite. The
           posterior cord is formed from the posterior divisions of all
           three trunks.

a **F**— The ventral rami which form its roots emerge behind the
           scalenus anterior muscle, between it and scalenus medius
           muscle.
b **T**— The cords are named according to their arrangement
           around the middle part of this artery.
c **F**— All the extensor muscles of the upper limb are supplied by
           the posterior cord.
d **F**— Latissimus dorsi is supplied by the thoracodorsal nerve
           which arises from the posterior cord.
e **T**— Through the medial and lateral pectoral nerves.

a **T**— By two heads, the short to the coracoid process and the
           long to the supraglenoid tubercle.
b **T**— The tendon of the long head lies in the shoulder joint
           surrounded by a synovial sheath in the intertubercular
           groove.
c **F**— Its distal attachment is to the radial tuberosity and by the
d **F**   bicipital aponeurosis to the deep fascia of the medial side
           of the forearm.
e **F**— It is a powerful spinator of the forearm and flexor at the
           elbow and shoulder joints.

155   The triceps muscle:
a   is attached to the infraglenoid tubercle of the scapula.   (   )
b   is attached to the borders of the radial groove of the humerus.   (   )
c   is attached to the ulnar olecranon.   (   )
d   acts mainly at the shoulder joint.   (   )
e   is supplied by the median nerve.   (   )

156   The brachial artery:
a   lies medial to biceps.   (   )
b   can be palpated over most of its course.   (   )
c   ends at the lower border of teres major by dividing into radial and ulnar arteries.   (   )
d   is crossed by the median cubital vein.   (   )
e   is crossed by the median nerve.   (   )

157   The musculocutaneous nerve:
a   is a terminal branch of the posterior cord of the brachial plexus.   (   )
b   descends in the arm between biceps and brachialis.   (   )
c   supplies coracobrachialis.   (   )
d   supplies cutaneous branches to the radial side of the forearm.   (   )
e   ends up as the medial cutaneous nerve of the forearm.   (   )

158   The radial nerve:
a   is a terminal branch of the posterior cord of the brachial plexus.   (   )
b   lies posterior to the humerus between the medial and lateral heads of triceps.   (   )
c   passes anterior to the elbow joint.   (   )
d   supplies the skin of the medial and anterior aspect of the forearm.   (   )
e   supplies the supinator muscle.   (   )

a **T**— Proximally it is attached by three heads to (a) and (b), and the lower part of the posterior aspect of the humerus
b **T** below the radial groove.

c **T**— Distally all its fibres are attached by a strong tendon to the olecranon.
d **F**— It is mainly an extensor at the elbow joint.
e **F**— It is supplied by the radial nerve.

a **T**— Throughout its course it lies medial to biceps covered only
b **T** by skin and fascia.
c **F**— It usually ends in the cubital fossa by dividing into radial and ulnar arteries.
d **T**— At its termination, but separated by the bicipital aponeurosis from the vein.
e **T**— The nerve accompanies the artery crossing anteriorly from lateral to medial in the mid upper arm.

a **F**— It is a terminal branch of the lateral cord of the brachial plexus.
b **T**— It then emerges lateral to these muscles and pierces the deep fascia in front of the elbow.
c **T**— It gives muscular branches to this muscle, biceps and brachialis.
d **T**— It ends as the lateral cutaneous nerve of the forearm and supplies both surfaces of the radial side of the forearm.
e **F**

a **T**— Arising as a branch of the posterior cord it descends obliquely through the posterior compartment between
b **T** these two heads of triceps. It then pierces the lateral intermuscular septum and lies anterior to the lateral epicondyle.
c **T**— Lying between brachialis medially and brachioradialis laterally.
d **F**— It supplies branches to triceps, brachioradialis and extensor carpi radialis longus, and to the skin of the lateral and posterior aspects of the arm and forearm by the lower lateral cutaneous nerve of arm and the posterior cutaneous nerve of forearm.
e **F**— This is supplied by the posterior interosseous nerve.

159 The median nerve:
a arises in the neck from the brachial plexus. ( )

b lies lateral to the axillary artery. ( )
c crosses the brachial artery. ( )

d has no muscular branches in the arm. ( )
e lies anterior to the biceps. ( )

160 The ulnar nerve:
a is a terminal branch of the medial cord of the brachial plexus. ( )
b descends to the elbow in the anterior compartment of the arm. ( )
c descends with the long hand of the triceps. ( )

d lies behind the medial epicondyle. ( )
e supplies branches to coracobrachialis. ( )

161 The radius:
a possesses a head which articulates with the scaphoid and lunate. ( )
b gives attachment to the biceps. ( )
c gives attachment to the triceps tendon. ( )

d possesses a palpable styloid process. ( )

e is attached to the ulna throughout the length of its interosseous border. ( )

162 The ulna:
a gives attachment to the brachialis muscle. ( )

b possesses a styloid process on the anteromedial surface of its lower end. ( )
c articulates at its lower end with an articular disc. ( )

d is palpable over the whole length of its posterior border. ( )
e is related inferiorly to the extensor carpi radialis muscle. ( )

a **F**— It is formed in the axilla from the medial and lateral cords of the brachial plexus.

b **T**

c **T**— Lying at first on its lateral side and then crosses the artery halfway down the arm to gain its medial side.

d **T**

e **F**— It lies medial to biceps and anterior to brachialis and triceps.

a **T**— It runs initially in the anterior compartment on the medial side of the upper arm then pierces the medial

b **F** intermuscular septum and continues in the posterior compartment.

c **F**— After piercing the medial intermuscular septum it descends between the septum and the medial head of triceps.

d **T**— At this point it is subcutaneous.

e **F**— It has no branches in the upper arm. Coracobrachialis is supplied by the musculocutaneous nerve.

a **F**— The head articulates with the capitulum of the humerus and the radial notch of the ulna.

b **T**— At the radial tuberosity.

c **F**— Triceps is attached to the olecranon of the ulna. Biceps is attached to the radial tuberosity of the radius.

d **T**— The styloid process, the lower end of the radius, and the radial head are all palpable.

e **T**— The fibrous interosseous membrane connects the adjacent interosseous borders of the radius and ulna.

a **T**— Brachialis is attached to the coronoid process of the upper end of the ulna.

b **F**— The small conical styloid process lies on the posteromedial side of the head of the ulna.

c **T**— The lower end, or head, articulates both with the lower end of the radius and with the articular disc which takes origin from the base of the ulnar styloid process.

d **T**— Together with the posterior part of the olecranon, the head and the styloid process.

e **F**— The extensor carpi ulnaris lies in the groove between the head and the styloid process.

163 **The cubital fossa:**
a is a quadrilateral space situated in front of the elbow joint. ( )

b is floored by the bicipital aponeurosis. ( )

c contains the median nerve. ( )
d contains the radial nerve. ( )

e is crossed by the medial cutaneous nerve of the forearm. ( )

164 **The elbow joint:**
a is lined by synovial membrane which is continuous with that of the superior radio-ulnar joint. ( )
b is strengthened by radial and ulnar collateral ligaments. ( )

c is strengthened by an ulnar collateral ligament. ( )

d owes most of its stability to the close proximity of brachialis and triceps. ( )
e is supplied by the posterior interosseous nerve. ( )

165 **The proximal radio-ulnar joint:**
a is of the condyloid variety. ( )
b occurs between the head of the radius and the radial notch of the ulna. ( )
c is stabilised mainly by the surrounding capsular ligament of the elbow joint. ( )

d owes its stability mainly to the annular ligament. ( )

e is separated from the elbow joint by a fibrocartilaginous disc. ( )

a **F**— It is a triangular fossa bounded proximally by a line joining the two epicondyles of the humerus and distally by the pronator teres medially and the brachioradialis laterally.

b **F**— The bicipital aponeurosis is an extension from biceps tendon, and lies in the roof of the fossa. It gains attachment to the deep fascia over the medial side of the forearm and to the posterior border of the ulna.

c **T**— The median nerve is the most medial of the structures
d **T** passing through the fossa. The brachial artery, the prominent biceps tendon, and the radial and posterior interosseous nerves lie laterally in this order.

e **T**— It is also crossed by lateral cutaneous branches and cubital veins.

a **T**— The elbow joint is of the hinge variety.

b **T**— The radial collateral is a strong triangular ligament attached to the lateral epicondyle proximally and the annular ligament distally.

c **T**— The ulnar collateral radiates from the medial epicondyle proximally to the coronoid process and the olecranon.

d **F**— The most important factors in stabilising the joint are the shape of the bones and strong capsule.

e **T**— It is also supplied by branches of the radial, median, ulnar and musculocutaneous nerves.

a **F**— It is a synovial joint of the pivot variety.
b **T**— The radial notch and the annular ligament from an osseofascial ring which encircles the head of the radius.

c **F**— This capsular ligament is attached to the upper border of the annular ligament and does little to increase the stability of the radio-ulnar joint.

d **T**— This is narrower below than above and thus holds firmly the head of the adult radius. (Dislocation is more common in the child as the head of the radius has a less conical shape.)

e **F**— The proximal end of the radius articulates directly with the trochlea of the humerus.

166 The distal radio-ulnar joint:
a is a synovial joint of the pivot variety. ( )

b owes its stability mainly to the capsular ligament. ( )

c with the superior radio-ulnar joint allows both
supination and pronation to occur. ( )
d pronation is a powerful movement because of the
action of biceps. ( )
e is separated from the wrist joint by a
fibrocartilaginous disc. ( )

167 The interosseous membrane in the forearm:
a connects the radius and ulna. ( )

b gives attachment to both flexor and extensor
muscles. ( )
c has fibres directed downwards and laterally. ( )
d has little intrinsic strength. ( )

e is closely related to the termination of the brachial
artery. ( )

168 The anterior superficial group of forearm muscles:
a all arise from the anterior surface of the lateral
epicondyle of the humerus. ( )
b includes pronator teres. ( )

c are all supplied by branches of the median nerve. ( )

d may effect flexion at the elbow. ( )

e has attachment to the anterior surface of both the
radius and the ulna. ( )

a T— The head of the ulna articulates with the ulnar notch on the radius.

b F— This is usually weak. Stability is dependent on the articular disc which is attached to the styloid process of the ulna and the medial edge of the distal articular surface of the radius.

c T— These movements occur about an axis joining the centre of the radial head and the ulnar styloid process.

d F— Biceps is a supinator muscle, and in most people this is the stronger movement.

e T— The disc separates the two joint cavities.

a T— It is attached to the adjacent interosseous borders of these two bones.

b T— Both the deep flexor and deep extensor muscles gain attachment to it.

c F— Its fibres are directed downwards and medially.

d F— It is a strong membrane and thus a force transmitted upwards through the hand, as in punching, is transmitted to the elbow joint via the ulna as well as the head of the radius.

e F— But the anterior and posterior interosseous arteries are closely related.

a F— They have a common origin from the anterior surface of the medial epicondyle of the humerus.

b T— From radial to ulnar side, the muscles are pronator teres, flexor carpi radialis, palmaris longus, flexor digitorum superficialis and flexor carpi ulnaris.

c F— Flexor carpi ulnaris is supplied by the ulnar nerve whilst all others are supplied by the median nerve.

d T— Since all these muscles cross the elbow joint they produce weak elbow flexion in addition to their other actions in the forearm and hand.

e T— The pronator teres and the flexor digitorum superficialis are attached to both bones. The flexor carpi ulnaris is attached to the posterior subcutaneous border of the ulna.

169   The flexor digitorum superficialis muscle:
  a   arises from both radius and ulna.   ( )

  b   lies deep to the median nerve.   ( )

  c   has four tendons in the hand which encircle
      the corresponding tendons of flexor digitorum
      profundus in the fingers.   ( )
  d   is attached distally to the base of the distal phalanx
      of the fingers.   ( )
  e   has its middle and ring finger tendons placed
      anterior to those of the index and little, when deep
      to the flexor retinaculum.   ( )

170   The ulnar bursa:
  a   invests all but one of the tendons of the superficial
      and deep flexors in the forearm.   ( )
  b   begins deep to the flexor retinaculum.   ( )
  c   extends into the digital synovial sheaths around
      the tendons of all fingers.   ( )
  d   extends into the digital synovial sheath around
      the tendon of the little finger.   ( )

  e   does not usually communicate with the radial bursa. ( )

171   The brachioradialis muscle is:
  a   attached proximally to the lower third of the
      lateral supracondylar ridge of the humerus.   ( )

  b   attached distally to the dorsal aspect of the base
      of the 3rd metacarpal bone.   ( )

  c   a flexor of the elbow.   ( )
  d   a pronator of the forearm.   ( )

  e   supplied by the posterior interosseous nerve.   ( )

a **T**— It arises from the common flexor origin, the medial aspect of the coronoid process of the ulna, the anterior oblique line of the radius and a tendinous arch which lies between them.

b **F**— The median nerve passes deep to the tendinous arch and passes distally deep to the muscle.

c **T**— The four tendons diverge in the palm, one passing to each finger. Over the proximal phalanx the tendon splits, and passing dorsally, encircles the corresponding tendon of

d **F** flexor digitorum profundus. It then gains attachment to the sides of the middle phalanx.

e **T**— And the former are more likely to be damaged in lacerations of the front of the wrist.

a **T**— The common synovial sheath, the ulnar bursa, lies deep to the flexor retinaculum. It commences 2–3 cm above the

b **F** wrist and ends in the middle of the palm, except for a

c **F** medial prolongation which extends around the tendons of the little finger as far as the distal phalanx. The tendons in

d **T** the remaining fingers have separate digital synovial sheaths deep to the fibrous flexor sheaths. A part of these tendons in the palm has no synovial sheath.

e **T**— The radial bursa invests the tendon of flexor pollicis longus from above the wrist to the terminal phalanx.

a **F**— This is the attachment of the extensor carpi radialis longus. The brachioradialis is attached to the upper two-thirds of the ridge.

b **F**— This is the attachment of the extensor carpi radialis brevis. The brachioradialis is attached to the lateral aspect of the lower end of the radius.

c **T**— Most strongly in the mid-prone position.

d **T**— It may also supinate the forearm, depending on the position of the hand.

e **F**— This nerve supplies the forearm muscles attached to the common extensor origin. The brachioradialis and extensor radialis longus are supplied by the radial nerve.

172   The extensor digitorum muscle:
a   is attached proximally to the anterior aspect of the lateral epicondyle of the humerus.   (   )
b   covers the proximal phalanges by dorsal expansions of its four tendons.   (   )
c   is attached to the bases of the proximal phalanges of the four fingers.   (   )

d   has small tendinous slips to the dorsal expansion from the lumbrical and interosseous muscles.   (   ).
e   is supplied by the radial nerve.   (   )

173   The supinator muscle:
a   forms part of the floor of the cubital fossa.   (   )
b   is attached to the medial epicondyle of the humerus.   (   )
c   is attached to the proximal end of the ulna.   (   )
d   is attached to the proximal end of the radius.   (   )
e   is supplied by the ulnar nerve.   (   )

174   The abductor pollicis longus muscle:
a   is attached to the interosseous membrane.   (   )
b   tendon passes deep to both extensor carpi radialis longus and brevis.   (   )
c   is attached to the base of the proximal phalanx of the thumb.   (   )
d   produces extension at the thumb's carpometacarpal joint.   (   )
e   possesses a separate synovial sheath around its tendon.   (   )

a **T**— This is the common extensor origin.

b **T**— It divides just above the wrist into four tendons. As each tendon passes a metacarpophalangeal joint it forms a

c **F** triangular dorsal expansion covering the proximal phalanx. At the apex of the expansion (distally) the tendon reforms and then divides into three slips; the middle is attached to the base of the middle phalanx, the outer two slips pass distally and gain attachment to the base of the terminal phalanx.

d **T**— These small tendons influence movements at the metacarpophalangeal and interphalangeal joints.

e **F**— The muscle is supplied by the posterior interosseous nerve.

a **T**— It obliquely crosses the apex of the cubital fossa after emerging from deep to brachioradialis.

b **F**— It is attached below the common extensor origin on the lateral epicondyle.

c **T**— It is attached to the supinator crest of the ulna and the area in front of the crest.

d **T**— Ulnar and humeral heads are attached to the anterior surface of the proximal third of the radius.

e **F**— It is supplied by the posterior interosseous branch of the radial nerve.

a **T**— It is attached to the posterior surface of the ulna and radius and the intervening interosseous membrane.

b **F**— The tendon is superficial to both carpal extensors.

c **F**— Its tendon is attached to the radial side of the base of the first metacarpal.

d **T**— It produces abduction and extension at this joint.

e **T**— As it lies in the most lateral compartment of the extensor retinaculum.

175 **The extensor pollicis longus muscle:**
 a   is attached to the interosseous membrane.   (   )

 b   passes deep to the extensor retinaculum.   (   )
 c   has a synovial sheath common with that of
     extensor indicis.   (   )
 d   is attached to the base of the distal phalanx of
     the thumb.   (   )
 e   is supplied by the radial nerve.   (   )

176 **The anatomical snuff box:**
 a   is bounded anteriorly by the tendons of extensor
     pollicis longus and brevis.   (   )
 b   is bounded posteriorly by the tendon of abductor
     pollicis longus.   (   )
 c   overlies the scaphoid and trapezium.   (   )

 d   contains the tendons of extensors carpi radialis
     longus and brevis on its floor.   (   )
 e   contains the basilic vein in its roof.   (   )

177 **The radial artery:**
 a   passes superficial to brachioradialis.   (   )

 b   lies lateral to the radial nerve in the forearm.   (   )
 c   lies on the anterior surface of the lower end of
     the radius.   (   )
 d   passes between the two heads of the first
     dorsal interosseous muscle.   (   )

 e   terminates in the superficial palmar arch.   (   )

a **T**— It is attached to the posterior surface of the ulna and adjacent interosseous membrane distal to abductor pollicis longus.

b **T**— Its tendon descends deep to the extensor retinaculum,

c **F** grooving the medial side of the dorsal tubercle of the radius. It has its own synovial sheath.

d **T**— It extends the terminal phalanx.

e **F**— It is supplied by the posterior interosseous nerve.

a **F**— Its boundaries are — anteriorly, the tendons of abductor pollicis longus and extensor pollicis brevis, and posteriorly,

b **F** the tendon of extensor pollicis longus.

c **T**— Together with the radial styloid process, the wrist joint and the base of the first metacarpal bone.

d **T**— Together with the radial artery.

e **F**— The cephalic vein overlies the snuff box.

a **F**— It lies deep to brachioradialis in the early part of its course, and medial to the radial nerve.

b **F**— The radial nerve is on its lateral side.

c **T**— It is subcutaneous here and the pulse can usually be felt.

d **T**— It leaves the dorsum of the hand by passing between the two heads of this muscle and then the two heads of the adductor pollicis muscle.

e **F**— It ends in the deep palmar arch.

178 **The ulnar artery:**
a gives rise to the anterior interosseous artery. ( )
b lies deep to the muscles attached to the common
flexor origin. ( )

c lies medial to the ulnar nerve. ( )
d crosses superficial to the flexor retinaculum. ( )
e supplies the deep extensor muscles of the forearm. ( )

179 **The radial nerve, in the forearm and hand:**
a lies deep to brachioradialis. ( )

b reaches the dorsum of the hand by passing across
the lower end of the radius. (
c passes deep to the extensor retinaculum. (
d supplies the skin on the lateral aspect of the
dorsum of the hand and the dorsum of the
lateral four digits. (
e has no muscular branches. (

180 **The posterior interosseous nerve:**
a arises at the level of the elbow joint. (
b lies in close relationship with the upper end of
the ulna. (

c passes through the supinator muscle. (

d supplies all the extensor muscles. (

e supplies the elbow and wrist joints. (

a F— This is a branch of the common interosseous artery.

b T— Lying deep to these muscles it descends on flexor digitorum profundus with the ulnar nerve on its medial side.

c F— It is lateral to the nerve.

d T— Ending along the lateral side of the pisiform.

e T— It gives nutrient arteries to the radius and ulna, and by its posterior interosseous branch it supplies the deep extensor muscles in the forearm.

a T— It passes down the arm with the radial artery on its medial side throughout most of its length.

b T

c F— It passes superficial to the structure.

d F— It supplies the dorsum of the hand but usually only the lateral two and a half digits as far as the distal interphalangeal joints.

e F— Its posterior interosseous branch supplies most of the extensor muscles of the forearm.

a T— It arises from the radial nerve under cover of

b F brachioradialis at the level of the elbow joint and pierces supinator. It then curves laterally around the neck of the radius.

c T— It passes between the humeral and ulnar heads of the muscle.

d F— It supplies all but extensor carpi radialis longus which is supplied by the radial nerve directly. Injury to the nerve produces wrist drop.

e T— Also the intercarpal joints.

181 **The median nerve in the forearm:**
  a passes between the heads of the pronator teres.   (   )

  b lies deep to flexor digitorum superficialis.   (   )

  c passes deep to the flexor retinaculum.   (   )
  d is a posterior relation of palmaris longus.   (   )

  e supplies all the forearm flexor muscles.   (   )

182 **The median nerve in the hand:**
  a supplies all the short muscles of the thumb.   (   )
  b supplies all the lumbrical muscles.   (   )

  c lies superficial to the flexor retinaculum.   (   )
  d terminates just distal to the flexor retinaculum.   (   )

  e supplies the palmar surface of the lateral three and a half digits.   (   )

183 **The ulnar nerve:**
  a is an anterior relation of the medial epicondyle of the humerus.   (   )
  b enters the forearm between the heads of the pronator teres.   (   )
  c lies on flexor digitorum profundus in the forearm.   (   )
  d supplies the ulnar half of the flexor digitorum sublimus.   (   )
  e supplies adductor pollicis.   (   )

184 **The ulnar nerve in the hand:**
  a passes into the hand deep to the flexor retinaculum.   (   )
  b supplies the dorsal surface of the medial two and a half fingers.   (   )
  c supplies all the interossei.   (   )
  d supplies abductor pollicis brevis.   (   )

  e supplies adductor pollicis.   (   )

a **T**— As it passes between the two heads of pronator teres it lies superficial to the ulnar artery, being separated from it by the deep head of the muscle.

b **T**— The nerve adheres to its deep surface but emerges lateral to its tendons above the wrist.

c **T**— Where it lies between the tendons of flexor carpi radialis

d **T** laterally and flexor superficialis medially. It lies deep to the palmaris longus tendon when this muscle is present.

e **F**— Flexor carpi ulnaris and the medial part of the flexor digitorum profundus are supplied by the ulnar nerve. The median nerve supplies the others.

a **F**— Adductor pollicis is supplied by the ulnar nerve.

b **F**— Only the lateral two lumbrical muscles are supplied by the median nerve.

c **F**— It passes deep to the flexor retinaculum in company with

d **T** the superficial and deep flexor tendons where it may become compressed.

e **T**— By palmar digital nerves which lie anterior to the digital arteries. These branches also innervate the nail beds and give articular branches to the joints of the fingers. The palmar branches supply the lateral two lumbrical muscles.

a **F**— It lies posterior to the epicondyle.

b **F**— This is the course of the medial nerve. The ulnar nerve lies between the heads of flexor carpi ulnaris.

c **T**— Deep to the flexor carpi ulnaris.

d **F**— In the forearm it supplies flexor carpi ulnaris and the ulnar half of flexor digitorum profundus.

e **T**— Also the hypothenar, interossei, and 3rd and 4th lumbrical muscles.

a **F**— It enters the hand superficially, anterior to the flexor retinaculum.

b **T**— By a dorsal cutaneous branch which divides into digital branches supplying these fingers as far as the distal interphalangeal joints.

c **T**— And the 3rd and 4th lumbricals.

d **F**— This muscle is supplied by the recurrent branch of the median nerve.

e **T**— The ulnar nerve supplies the adductor pollicis.

185 The carpal bones:

a   are arranged into proximal, middle and distal rows. (   )

b   which form the distal articular surface of the
wrist joint are the scaphoid, lunate and pisiform.   (   )

c   give attachment to the flexor retinaculum.   (   )

d   give attachment to the extensor retinaculum.   (   )

e   give attachment to the lumbrical muscles.   (   )

186 The metacarpal bone of:

a   the thumb gives attachment to the lateral
interossei muscles.   (   )

b   the thumb articulates with the trapezium.   (   )

c   the thumb gives attachment to flexor pollicis brevis. (   )

d   the index finger articulates with those of the
thumb and middle fingers.   (   )

e   the little finger articulates with the lunate.   (   )

187 The wrist joint:

a   comprises the lower articular surfaces of the
radius and ulna and the proximal row of carpal
bones.   (   )

b   usually communicates with the distal radio-ulnar
joint.   (   )

c   owes its stability to the neighbouring tendons.   (   )

d   is an ellipsoid joint.   (   )

e   contributes the major degree of flexion at the wrist. (   )

a F— They are arranged as a proximal row of three bones, the scaphoid, lunate and triquetral; a distal row of four, the trapezium, trapezoid, capitate and hamate; and an anteromedially situated pisiform.

b F— This surface comprises from lateral to medial, the scaphoid, lunate and triquetral.

c T— The flexor retinaculum extends from the pisiform and hamate bones medially to the scaphoid and trapezium laterally.

d T— The extensor retinaculum extends from the distal end of the radius to the medial side of the carpus, i.e. the pisiform, triquetral and hamate.

e F— These unite the long digital flexor and extensor tendons.

a T— Together with the opponens pollicis and abductor pollicis longus muscles.

b T— Its articular surface is saddle-shaped.

c F— Flexor pollicis brevis is attached to the flexor retinaculum and the base of the proximal phalanx of the thumb.

d F— The 1st metacarpal, unlike the 3rd metacarpal, has no articulation with the index finger; (b) and (d) increase the mobility of the thumb.

e F— The 5th metacarpal articulates with the hamate.

a F— The lower end of the radius and the fibrocartilaginous disc overlying the head of the ulna articulate with the proximal row of carpal bones. Only on rare occasions when this disc

b F is perforated does the wrist joint communicate with the distal radio-ulnar joint.

c T— Together with the capsular and the medial and lateral collateral ligaments which strengthen it. The shapes of the bones contribute minimally.

d T— This permits flexion, extension, adduction (ulnar deviation), abduction (radial deviation) and circumduction. No rotation occurs.

e F— Wrist movements take place at the radiocarpal (wrist joint), midcarpal and carpometacarpal joints. The midcarpal has particular effect in flexion and abduction.

188   The metacarpophalangeal joints:
a   are synovial joints of the hinge variety.   (   )

b   of the medial four digits are bound together.   (   )

c   may be abducted by the dorsal interossei muscle.   (   )

d   may be adducted by the palmar interossei muscles.   (   )

e   may be flexed by the lumbricals.   (   )

189   The palmar aponeurosis:
a   is strengthened deep fascia.   (   )

b   is firmly attached to the palmar skin.   (   )
c   is continuous proximally with the flexor retinaculum.   (   )
d   distally is continuous with the long flexor tendons.   (   )
e   is attached distally to the deep transverse
    ligament of the palm.   (   )

190   The flexor retinaculum:
a   is attached to the lower end of the radius.   (   )
b   is attached to the lower end of the ulna.   (   )
c   is attached to the pisiform bone.   (   )
d   gives origin to the thenar and hypothenar muscles.   (   )
e   overlies all tendons, arteries and nerves
    proceeding to the palm.   (   )

191   The palmar muscle spaces:
a   are two in number.   (   )
b   are each deep to the palmar aponeurosis.   (   )
c   are separated by intermuscular septa.   (   )
d   contain the thenar muscles laterally.   (   )
e   contain the lumbrical muscles centrally.   (   )

a F— They are ellipsoid joints, allowing movement in two planes at right angles to each other, and circumduction.
b T— By an extension of the strong palmar thickenings of these joints forming the deep transverse ligaments of the palm.
c T— And by abductor pollicis longus and brevis and abductor digiti minimi in the case of the thumb and little finger respectively.
d T— And by adductor pollicis in the case of the thumb. Thumb movements of abduction and adduction occur at the carpometacarpal joint.
e T— The attachment of these muscles to both long flexor and extensor tendons flex the metacarpophalangeal but extend the interphalangeal joints.

a T— It comprises the strong central, triangular part of the deep fascia.
b T— And its apex is continuous with the flexor retinaculum. Its
c T   base divides distally into four slips which bifurcate around
d F   the long flexor tendons, gaining attachment to the fibrous
e T   flexor digital sheaths and to the deep transverse ligaments of the palm.

a F— It is a thickening of deep fascia gaining attachment to the carpal
b F   bones, medially to the pisiform and hamate, laterally to the
c T   scaphoid and trapezium.
d T
e F— The ulnar artery and nerve and the palmar branches of the median and ulnar nerves all cross it superficially. The median nerve lies deep to it.

a F— There are three palmar muscle spaces separated by two
b F   septa which pass deeply from the lateral and medial margins
c T   of the palmar aponeurosis to the shafts of the 1st and 5th
d T   metacarpal bones. The lateral space containing the thenar
e T   muscles, and the medial, containing the hypothenar muscles, are covered superficially by the deep fascia of the palm. The central space, containing the long flexor tendons and lumbrical muscles, deep and superficial palmar arches and the median and ulnar nerves, is covered by the palmar aponeurosis.

192   The fibrous flexor digital sheaths:
a   are modifications of the deep fascia of the fingers.   (   )
b   are attached to the phalanges.   (   )
c   proximally, are continuous with the palmar
        aponeurosis.   (   )

d   overlie the first phalanges only.   (   )

e   enclose the tendons of flexor digitorum profundus
        only.   (   )

193   The muscles of the thenar eminence:
a   are all attached to the radial side of the flexor
        retinaculum.   (   )
b   are all supplied by the radial nerve.   (   )

c   have abductor pollicis brevis lying most
        superficially.   (   )
d   are all attached distally to the first metacarpal bone. (   )
e   have an attachment to the base of the distal
        phalanx of the thumb.   (   )

194   The interossei muscles:
a   are eight in total.   (   )
b   all arise by two heads from adjacent metacarpal
        bones.   (   )

c   are all attached distally to the base of the
        corresponding proximal phalanx and the dorsal
        extensor expansion.   (   )
d   may flex the metacarpophalangeal joints.   (   )
e   may extend the middle and distal phalanges.   (   )

a T— Here the deep fascia is modified, forming these fibrous
b T   sheaths which make osseofascial tunnels by arching over
c T   the tendons and gaining attachment to the sides of the
        phalanges. Proximally they are continuous with the palmar
        aponeurosis.
d F— Each extends to the base of the distal phalanx and is lined
        with synovial membrane.
e F— Both the long flexor tendons, superficialis and profundus,
        are enclosed within these sheaths.

a T— And to its bony attachments.

b F— The recurrent branch of the median nerve supplies all of
        them.

c T— Opponens pollicis and flexor pollicis brevis lie deep to the
        short abductor of the thumb.
d F— Both abductor pollicis brevis and flexor pollicis brevis are
e F   attached to the base of the proximal phalanx of the thumb.
        The opponens is attached to the body of the 1st
        metacarpal bone. (N.B. The adductor pollicis, supplied by
        the ulnar nerve, is not a muscle of the thenar eminence,
        though it is a short muscle of the thumb.)

a T— There are four dorsal and four palmar muscles.
b F— These muscles are attached to the bodies of the metacarpal
        bones, the palmar by a single head and the dorsal by two
        heads, from adjacent sides of the metacarpal bones.
c T— Their main action is at the metacarpophalangeal joints
        producing adduction (palmar) and abduction (dorsal). They
        may also assist flexion at these joints.
d T
e T— By their attachment to the extensor expansion they help
        the lumbricals to extend the middle and distal phalanges.

195 The lumbrical muscles:
a   are each attached to a tendon of flexor digitorum
superficialis.   (   )
b   have each a tendon winding round the ulnar side
of the corresponding metacarpophalangeal joint.   (   )

c   are all supplied by the median nerve.   (   )

d   produce flexion at the metacarpophalangeal joints
of the finger.   (   )
e   produce flexion at the interphalangeal joints.   (   )

196 In the veins of the upper limb the:
a   cephalic vein has no valves.   (   )
b   the cephalic vein crosses the anatomical snuff box.   (   )
c   basilic vein commences at the medial aspect of
the palmar venous arch.   (   )

d   basilic vein pierces the clavipectoral fascia.   (   )

e   median cubital vein lies deep to the bicipital
aponeurosis.   (   )

197 Lymph drainage of the upper limb:
a   comprises a superficial and a deep group of
vessels and nodes.   (   )

b   has no lymph nodes distal to the axilla.   (   )
c   is entirely to the axillary groups of lymph nodes.   (   )

d   deeper tissues drain to the pectoral group of nodes. (   )

e   is eventually into the internal jugular vein.   (   )

a **F**— Each is attached to a tendon of flexor digitorum profundus.

b **F**— The tendons pass round the radial side of the joints and are attached distally to the base of the proximal phalanx and into the fibrous extensor expansion.

c **F**— The radial two muscles are supplied by the median nerve and the ulnar two by the ulnar nerve.

d **T**— They extend the interphalangeal joints. When paralysed, there is a resulting claw-hand, partial or complete.

e **F**

a **F**— Numerous valves are found in the majority of upper limb veins.

b **T**

c **F**— The superficial venous arch lies dorsally, the basilic vein arising medially. The cephalic vein, arising laterally, approximates in position to the pre-axial border of the fetal limb.

d **F**— The basilic vein pierces the deep fascia just proximal to the elbow joint. The cephalic vein pierces the clavipectoral fascia.

e **F**— The vein is superficial to the aponeurosis which separates the vein from the brachial artery. The median cubital vein is often used for intravenous injections so the arterial relations are of clinical importance.

a **T**— The superficial vessels drain the skin and related structures and follow the large superficial veins. The deep vessels drain the muscles, bones and joints, and follow the deep vessels.

b **F**— A cubital node is sited posterior to the medial epicondyle.

c **T**— These are arranged in five regions of the axilla: pectoral, lateral, subscapular, central and apical nodes.

d **F**— Deeper tissues drain first to the lateral group of nodes and then to central and apical nodes. The pectoral nodes drain the tissues of the anterior chest wall, including the mammary gland.

e **T**— The apical nodes drain the other nodes and are continuous with the infraclavicular group of nodes. From the latter, lymph trunks emerge and drain into the internal jugular vein.

198   In the nerve supply of the upper limb:
a the skin over the thumb is supplied by the
    C6 dermatome.   ( )
b an injury to the lower trunk of the brachial
    plexus produces a characteristic clawed hand.   ( )
c damage to the radial nerve in the radial groove
    produces wrist drop.   ( )
d injury to the median nerve at the wrist produces
    loss of sensation of the front of the thumb, index
    and middle fingers.   ( )
e injury to the axillary nerve produces impaired
    abduction of the humerus.   ( )

VII The Lower Limb

199   In the development of the lower limb:
a the axial artery arises from the superior vesical
    artery.   ( )

b lateral rotation of the limb occurs between the hip
    and knee regions.   ( )
c the muscles supplied by the posterior divisions of
    the ventral rami have been carried on to the
    anterolateral aspect of the limb.   ( )

d synovial joints are present between some of the
    bones of the pelvic girdle.   ( )

e the posterior division of the anterior primary rami
    of L2, 3 and 4 give rise to the obturator nerve.   ( )

200   The ilium:
a gives attachment to the gluteus maximus muscles
    between the middle and posterior gluteal lines.   ( )
b is bordered posteriorly by the lesser sciatic notch.   ( )
c gives attachment to the rectus femoris muscle
    anteroinferiorly.   ( )
d has a secondary centre of ossification appearing
    along its upper border at puberty.   ( )
e gives attachment to sartorius.   ( )

a **T**— The little finger is supplied by C8.

b **T**— This is due to paralysis of the small muscles of the hand and of the long digital flexors.

c **T**— Due to paralysis of the long digital and carpal extensors.

d **T**— Also paralysis of the thenar muscles and the 1st and 2nd lumbricals.

e **T**— Due to paralysis of the deltoid, there is also loss of sensation over the attachment of this muscle.

a **F**— The axial artery is represented by part of the internal iliac artery and its inferior gluteal branch. The artery roughly follows the course of the adult sciatic nerve. The superior vesical artery is a derivative of the fetal umbilical artery.

b **F**— Medial rotation occurs, so that the plantar surface of the foot is directed backwards, and later downwards.

c **T**— They are innervated by the femoral and common peroneal nerves. The large muscles of the lower limb are used mainly in locomotion. When standing upright, the weight is carried by bones and ligaments.

d **T**— The sacro-iliac joint is synovial but becomes increasingly fibrosed in later life. The two pubic bones are united by a symphysis. In these joints movement is minimal. The ilium, ischium and pubis have cartilaginous joints and no movement occurs.

e **F**— This is the derivation of the femoral nerve, the obturator is derived from the anterior divisions of the same roots.

a **F**— This is the area of attachment of the gluteus medius muscle.

b **F**— The greater sciatic notch forms the posterior border.

c **T**— The reflected head is attached to this area above the acetabulum.

d **T**— The iliac crest epiphysis fuses about the 20th year.

e **T**— At the anterior superior iliac spine.

201   The obturator foramen:

a   is bounded posteriorly by the iliac part of the
acetabulum.   (   )

b   transmits the inferior gluteal nerve.   (   )

c   is separated from the pudendal nerve by the
obturator internus muscle.   (   )

d   transmits the obturator artery and nerve.   (   )

e   transmits the superior gluteal artery.   (   )

202   The greater trochanter of the femur:

a   is united anteriorly to the lesser trochanter by the
intertrochanteric line.   (   )

b   gives attachment to the piriformis muscle along
its upper border.   (   )

c   gives attachment to the quadratus femoris muscle.   (   )

d   gives attachment to the gluteus minimus muscle
along its anterior border.   (   )

e   gives attachment to the gluteus maximus along its
posterior border.   (   )

203   The lesser trochanter of the femur:

a   gives attachment to the pectineus muscle.   (   )

b   gives attachment to iliacus.   (   )

c   gives attachment to the flexors at the hip joint.   (   )

d   gives attachment to vastus intermedius.   (   )

e   has a secondary centre of ossification which
appears in the 10th year and fuses in the 18th year.   (   )

204   The body of the femur:

a   forms an angle of about 125° with the neck.   (   )

b   gives attachment to the gluteus maximus muscle
along the linea aspera.   (   )

c   has no muscles attached to its anterior surface.   (   )

d   gives attachment to the short head of biceps.   (   )

e   gives attachment to adductor brevis.   (   )

a **F**— The ilium forms no part of the foramen, which is bounded by the ischium and pubis.
b **F**— The inferior gluteal nerve passes through the greater sciatic foramen.
c **T**— The pudendal canal is related to the medial surface of this muscle.
d **T**— The obturator vessels and nerve pass in the obturator groove and, through the foramen, into the thigh. The nerve supplies the adductor group of muscles.
e **F**— The superior gluteal vessels and nerve pass through the greater sciatic foramen.

a **T**— The intertrochanteric crest joins the structures posteriorly.
b **T**— Obturator internus and externus are attached to its medial surface.
c **F**— This muscle is attached to the quadrate tubercle on the intertrochanteric crest.
d **T**— And the gluteus medius is attached diagonally to the lateral surface.
e **F**— The femoral attachment of this muscle is to the gluteal tuberosity.

a **F**— This muscle is attached to the body of the bone below the lesser trochanter.
b **T**— Iliacus joins with psoas and is attached to the lesser trochanter and to the bone just below.
c **T**— Psoas is also a medial rotator.
d **F**— This muscle is attached to the anterior surface of the body of the femur.
e **T**— Centres for the head (1yr) and greater trochanter (5yrs) also unite with the body at this time.

a **T**— This is less in the female. The body is inclined medially at an angle of about 20° with the vertical.
b **F**— This muscle is attached to the gluteal tuberosity between the linea aspera and the quadrate tubercle.
c **F**— The vastus intermedius has a wide attachment from this area.
d **T**— Along the linea aspera in the middle of the body.
e **T**— Along the proximal part of the linea aspera.

205   The lower end of the femur:
   a   gives attachment to the adductor magnus.   ( )

   b   gives attachment to the lateral ligament of the
knee joint on the lateral epicondyle.   ( )

   c   gives attachment to the plantaris muscle in a pit
below the lateral epicondyle.   ( )

   d   gives attachment to the patellar ligament.   ( )

   e   has a secondary centre of ossification which
unites with the body in the 20th year.   ( )

206   The capsule of the hip joint:
   a   is attached along the intertrochanteric crest.   ( )

   b   is attached along the intertrochanteric line.   ( )

   c   carries blood vessels to the head of the femur.   ( )

   d   is thickened inferiorly as the iliofemoral ligament.   ( )

   e   limits flexion at the hip joint.   ( )

207   In movements at the hip joint:
   a   abduction is produced mainly by the gluteus
medius and minimus muscles.   ( )

   b   medial rotation is produced by gluteus medius
and minimus.   ( )

   c   extension is limited by tension in the three
capsular thickenings.   ( )

   d   lateral rotation is largely performed by muscles
supplied by the femoral nerve.   ( )

   e   flexion is produced by muscles supplied by the
femoral nerve.   ( )

a **T**— To the medial supracondylar line ending below at the adductor tubercle.

b **T**— Also the medial epicondyle gives attachment to the medial ligament.

c **F**— This is the point of attachment of the popliteus muscle.

d **F**— The tendon is attached to the tibial tuberosity.

e **T**— It appears in the 8th–9th month of intra-uterine life and is an indication of fetal maturity.

a **F**— The posterior attachment is to the neck about 1 cm proximal to the crest.

b **T**

c **T**— In the retinacular fibres of the capsule. Fractures across the neck heal poorly when these vessels are torn.

d **F**— This powerful Y-shaped ligament passes anteriorly from the anterior inferior iliac spine to the intertrochanteric line.

e **F**— The strong iliofemoral and the other capsular ligaments tighten and stabilise the joint in extension. Active flexion is limited because of the attachments of the muscles and is further limited if the knee joint is in the extended position.

a **T**— Abduction on the grounded leg is important in walking, as in it the opposite hip bone is raised, thus allowing the opposite limb to swing forwards clear of the ground.

b **T**— The iliopsoas muscle is also involved.

c **T**— These three ligaments spiral in such a way as to all limit this movement.

d **F**— This movement is performed by gluteus maximus and the short posterior articular muscles, supplied by nerves emerging through the greater sciatic notch. The femoral nerve supplies mainly the extensor muscles at the knee joint.

e **T**— Rectus femoris and sartorius are supplied by the nerve. Iliopsoas, the main flexor, is supplied by femoral and direct branches from the 12th thoracic and upper 4 lumbar nerves.

208   The hip joint is directly related:
   a   anteriorly to the psoas bursa.   (   )

   b   superiorly to the gluteus medius muscle.   (   )

   c   posteriorly to the sciatic nerve.   (   )

   d   inferiorly to the obturator externus muscle. (   )

   e   to the femoral nerve.   (   )

209   The gluteus maximus muscle:
   a   is attached to the sacrospinous ligament.   (

   b   is attached to the iliotibial tract.   (

   c   is supplied by the superior gluteal nerve. (

   d   overlies the lesser sciatic foramen.   (

   e   abducts the hip joint.   (

**210   The greater sciatic foramen transmits the
       nerves supplying the:**
   a   tensor fascia lata muscle.   (   )
   b   gluteal muscles.   (   )
   c   hamstring muscles.   (   )
   d   adductor muscles.   (   )

   e   perineal muscles.   (   )

a T— The bursa frequently communicates with the joint through a hole in the capsule between the iliofemoral and pubofemoral ligaments.
b F— This muscle overlaps the gluteus minimus and the reflected head of the rectus femoris muscle which separate it from the joint.
c F— The nerve is separated from the joint by the obturator internus and quadratus femoris muscles but its proximity to the joint has important surgical implications.
d T— The close proximity of all the above muscles contribute to the marked stability of the joint.
e F— The nerve lies on psoas and iliacus.

a F— Its upper attachment includes the sacrotuberous ligament, the ilium, the sacrum and the coccyx.
b T— Through which it stabilises the knee joint and produces extension at the joint.
c F— The superior nerve does not contribute. The muscle is supplied by the inferior gluteal nerve.
d T— Also the greater sciatic foramen and the vessels, nerves and muscles these foramen transmit.
e F— It is the main extensor at the hip joint.

a T— The superior gluteal nerve emerges above piriformis and
b T   also supplies gluteus medius and minimus muscles.
c T— The sciatic nerve emerges below the piriformis.
d F— The adductor muscles are innervated by the obturator nerve which passes through the obturator foramen.
e T— The pudendal nerve emerges below the piriformis, hooks around the ischial spine and passes through the lesser sciatic foramen into the pudendal canal on the lateral wall of the ischiorectal fossa.

211   The semimembranosus muscle:
   a   is attached superiorly to the ischial tuberosity.   (   )
   b   is attached distally to the medial aspect of the body
       of the tibia behind the attachment of the gracilis
       tendon.   (   )
   c   has a recurrent tendinous expansion on to the lateral
       femoral condyle.   (   )
   d   has a separate head attached to the linea aspera
       near the lateral lip and the upper part of the lateral
       supracondylar line of the femur.   (   )
   e   is supplied by the obturator nerve.   (   )

212   The sciatic nerve:
   a   is formed in the pelvis posterior to the fibres
       of the piriformis muscle.   (   )

   b   is directly related to the ischium.   (   )
   c   is directly related to the adductor magnus muscle.   (   )
   d   innervates part of the adductor magnus muscle.   (   )

   e   usually divides into its terminal branches just
       above the popliteal fossa.   (   )

213   The pectineus muscle:
   a   is attached to the upper part of the obturator
       membrane.   (   )
   b   is attached to the body of the femur.   (   )
   c   is supplied by the anterior division of the
       obturator nerve.   (   )

   d   lies in the same plane as the adductor longus
       muscle.   (   )

   e   is a medial rotator at the hip joint.   (   )

214   The adductor magnus:
   a   is attached to the anterior superior iliac spine.   (   )
   b   is attached to the lesser trochanter.   (   )
   c   is attached to the length of the linea aspera.   (   )
   d   is supplied by both the sciatic and obturator nerves.   (   )

   e   can extend the femur.   (   )

a T— The attachment is the most medial of the hamstrings.
b F— The tendon is attached in a groove on the posteromedial aspect of the tibial condyle proximal to the gracilis attachment.

c T— This is the oblique popliteal ligament.

d F— This describes the attachment of the short head of the biceps muscle.

e F— The innervation is from the sciatic.

a F— It is formed on the anterior surface of this muscle from the L4, 5 and S1, 2 and 3 nerves and leaves the pelvis through the greater sciatic foramen.
b T— Then passing on to obturator internus and quadratus
c T femoris muscles which separate it from the hip joint.
d T— It descends between this muscle and the hamstrings and innervates the part of the adductor magnus attached to the ischial tuberosity.
e T— Having supplied the hamstring muscles and the hamstring part of the adductor magnus muscle.

a F— It is attached to the superior aspect of the pubic bone.

b T— Along a line joining the lesser trochanter to the linea aspera.
c F— The obturator nerve is a posterior relation and supplies gracilis, adductor longus and adductor brevis. Pectineus is supplied by branches of the femoral nerve.
d T— Obturator externus and adductor brevis muscles separate the pectineus and adductor longus in front from adductor magnus muscle behind.
e T— Also a weak flexor.

a F— Proximally it is attached to the outer surface of the ischiopubic
b T ramus, distally to the linea aspera, the medial supracondylar
c T line and the adductor tubercle.
d T— Branches from the sciatic nerve supply the ischial part of the muscle. The remainder is supplied by the obturator nerve.
e T— In addition to adducting it.

215   **The obturator nerve:**
   a   is a branch of the upper part of the lumbosacral plexus. ( )
   b   enters the thigh through the obturator groove. ( )

   c   anterior division descends between the adductor longus and the adductor magnus. ( )
   d   posterior division pierces the obturator internus muscle. ( )
   e   supplies the pectineus muscle. ( )

216   **The sartorius muscle:**
   a   is attached to the anterior inferior iliac spine. ( )
   b   forms the medial boundary of the femoral triangle. ( )

   c   is an extensor at the knee and hip joints. ( )

   d   roofs in the femoral vessels in the mid-thigh. ( )
   e   is supplied by branches of the anterior divisions of the lumbar plexus. ( )

217   **The rectus femoris muscle:**
   a   forms part of the quadriceps muscle. ( )

   b   gains attachment from the lateral lip of the linea aspera. ( )
   c   has a superior attachment to the anterior inferior iliac spine. ( )
   d   has lower medial fibres that run almost horizontally to the patella. ( )

   e   is partly supplied by the obturator nerve. ( )

138

a **T**— It arises from the anterior divisions of L2, L3 and L4.

b **T**— The nerve divides into anterior and posterior divisions at this point. The groove is bounded by the pubis, ischium and obturator membrane.

c **F**— It lies between the adductor longus and brevis.

d **F**— It pierces the obturator externus and lies between adductor brevis and magnus.

e **F**— This muscle is supplied by the femoral nerve.

a **F**— It is attached to the anterior superior iliac spine.

b **F**— It forms the lateral boundary. It also serves to separate the adductor muscles at the hip superomedially from the extensor muscles at the knee inferolaterally.

c **F**— It is a flexor and its actions are best demonstrated by sitting in the crossed leg position, hence its synonym, the tailor's muscle.

d **T**— They lie in the adductor canal.

e **F**— The femoral nerve (from the posterior divisions) usually supplies it.

a **T**— The quadriceps muscle mass also includes the three vastus muscles, and is a powerful extensor at the knee joint.

b **F**— The rectus has no attachment to the femur. The vastus muscles have extensive attachments to this bone.

c **T**— And a reflected head to the ilium just above the acetabulum.

d **F**— These fibres are part of the vastus medialis muscle, and prevent the patella moving too far laterally during extension.

e **F**— It is supplied by the femoral nerve.

218   The femoral triangle:
  a is bounded medially by the adductor longus muscle. ( )

  b is bounded laterally by the rectus femoris muscle. ( )
  c contains an extension of the transversalis fascia. ( )

  d contains both the femoral artery and its vein. ( )

  e has a defect in its fascial roof. ( )

219   The femoral artery:
  a is formed behind the midpoint of the inguinal ligament. ( )

  b has the femoral nerve on its lateral side in the femoral triangle. ( )
  c in the adductor canal has vastus medialis situated anterolaterally to it. ( )
  d lies posterior to sartorius. ( )
  e leaves the thigh by passing inferior to the adductor magnus tendon. ( )

220   The femoral vein:
  a passes anterior to the upper attachment of the) pectineus muscle. ( )
  b is separated by the femoral canal from the lacunar part of the inguinal ligament. ( )
  c lies anterior to its artery in the adductor canal. ( )

  d passes through a separate opening in the adductor magnus from the artery. ( )

  e has the saphenous nerve lying medially in the adductor canal. ( )

a T— The muscle also forms part of the floor of the triangle along with pectineus and iliopsoas muscles.

b F— Sartorius forms the lateral boundary.

c T— This fascia and the fascia of iliacus are continued beneath the inguinal ligament as the femoral sheath.

d T— The vein lies medially and can enlarge into the femoral canal on its medial side. These are important surgical relations.

e T— The saphenous opening in the deep fascia is traversed by the great saphenous vein and is an important landmark in vein surgery. The opening lies 3 cm below and 1 cm lateral to the pubic tubercle.

a F— The surface marking lies medial to this at the midinguinal point (midway between the anterior superior iliac spine and the symphysis pubis). The inferior epigastric artery thus forms a medial relation of the deep inguinal ring, which is situated above the midpoint of the inguinal ligament.

b T— The iliopsoas separates both structures from the hip joint.

c T— The artery lies at first on adductor longus and then adductor magnus.

d T— The sartorius forms the roof of the adductor canal.

e F— It passes through an opening in the muscle about 10 cm above the knee joint and becomes the popliteal artery.

a T— Then descends on adductor longus.

b T— The femoral canal is the space through which femoral herniae may develop.

c F— The vein passes from the medial to the posterior aspect of the artery.

d F— They are closely related in the adductor canal and pass through the single opening. The popliteal vein lies posterior to the popliteal artery.

e T— The nerve then passes medially to join the great saphenous vein in the lower leg.

221   The femoral nerve:
a is formed from the anterior divisions of the lumbar 2, 3 and 4 roots.   (   )
b is enclosed in the lateral part of the femoral sheath. (   )

c lies in the groove between iliacus and psoas as it passes deep to the inguinal ligament.   (   )
d branches are divided into superficial and deep by the medial circumflex femoral artery.   (   )

e has a saphenous branch which enters the popliteal space with the femoral vessels.   (   )

222   The patella:
a ossifies in mesenchyme.   (   )

b has a larger lateral than medial articular facet.   (   )
c receives tendinous expansions from vastus lateralis muscle on its lateral border.   (   )
d receives muscular attachments from the vastus medialis along its medial border.   (   )

e gives attachment to gracilis along its medial surface. (   )

223   The upper end of the tibia:
a has a prominent tibial tuberosity on its superior surface.   (   )
b articulates with the lateral articular facet of the patella.   (   )
c gives attachment to the ends of the cartilaginous menisci along the intercondylar ridge.   (   )
d gives attachment to the semimembranosus muscle.   (   )

e has a centre of ossification which fuses with the body about the 20th year.   (   )

a **F**— These form the obturator nerve; the femoral arises from the posterior divisions of the same roots.

b **F**— The nerve is lateral to the artery but lies outside the sheath.

c **T**— It then divides into a number of terminal branches.

d **F**— The lateral circumflex femoral artery passes between the branches. The superficial branches are mainly cutaneous but there are branches to sartorius. The deeper branches are mainly muscular (to quadriceps femoris) but the saphenous nerve is sensory.

e **F**— The nerve leaves the adductor canal, passing under, sartorius to the medial side of the knee. It accompanies the great saphenous vein in the lower leg.

a **F**— It is a sesamoid bone ossifying in cartilage, a centre appearing in the 5th year.

b **T**— Both facets are further divided transversely.

c **T**— The retinacula. Further expansions pass to the upper border of the tibia.

d **T**— These fibres stabilise the patella during knee extension when there is a tendency for the patella to dislocate laterally.

e **F**— Gracilis is attached to the upper part of the medial surface of the tibia.

a **F**— The tuberosity is on the anterior border and receives the attachment of the patellar ligament.

b **F**— The patella articulates with the lower end of the femur.

c **T**—The cruciate ligaments are also attached to this ridge.

d **T**—The muscle is attached in a groove on the posteromedial aspect of the upper end.

e **T**— The centre appears about the 9th month of intra-uterine life.

224   The body of the tibia:
a   has the interosseous membrane attached to its
     posterior border.   (   )
b   has a prominent nutrient foramen in its upper third. (   )

c   gives attachment to flexor hallucis longus below
     the soleal line.   (   )
d   gives attachment to tibialis anterior over its lateral
     surface.   (   )
e   gives attachment to peroneus brevis on its
     mid-lateral surface.   (.)

225   The lower end of the tibia:
a   extends beyond the fibula.   (   )

b   is grooved posteromedially by the tendon of tibialis
     posterior.   (   )
c   is grooved anteromedially by the tibialis anterior.   (   )

d   unites with the body before the upper end.   (   )

e   gives attachment to the deltoid ligament.   (   )

226   The fibula:
a   gives attachment to the biceps tendon at the base
     of the head of the bone.   (   )
b   is related to the tibial nerve at its neck.   (   )
c   malleolar fossa is situated posteromedially at the
     lower end of the bone.   (   )
d   gives attachment to popliteus over its upper
     posterior surface.   (   )
e   upper and lower ends unite with the body about
     the same time as those of the tibia.   (   )

a F—The membrane is attached to the lateral border of the body.

b T— On the posterior surface just below the soleal line. However, much of its blood supply is from the muscles attached and through the periosteum. Absence of muscle attachments in the lower part of the tibia is a contributory factor to the poor healing of fractures in this region.

c F— This muscle is attached to the fibula. The tibia gives attachment to flexor digitorum longus and tibialis posterior.

d T— The medial surface is subcutaneous but gives attachment to the sartorius, gracilis and semitendinosus superiorly.

e F— This muscle is attached to the lower two-thirds of the lateral surface of the fibula.

a F— The tip of the lateral (fibular) malleolus extends distal to the medial tibial (malleolus).

b T— Lying medial to the tendon of flexor digitorum longus.

c F— The anterior border is smooth and is crossed by the tendons of the muscles in the anterior compartment of the leg.

d T— The secondary centre appears at 1 year and unites at 18 years.

e T— This medial ligament of the ankle joint is triangular in shape with its apex attached to the medial malleolus.

a T— The fibular collateral ligament is attached in front of the apex of the head.

b F— The common peroneal nerve is related at this site.

c T— It gives attachment to the posterior tibiofibular ligament and forms a useful marker when orientating the bone.

d F— The soleus muscle is attached to this area.

e T— 20 and 18 years respectively. The primary centres for the bodies of both bones appear about the 2nd month of intra-uterine life.

227   The knee joint:
a   is a condyloid joint.   (   )
b   has articular fibrocartilage covering the bony
    surfaces.   (   )
c   patella and femoral facets are in apposition except
    in full extension.   (   )
d   medial and lateral tibial articular surfaces are
    continuous with each other anteriorly.   (   )
e   medial and lateral femoral articular surfaces are
    continuous with each other anteriorly.   (   )

228   In the knee joint the:
a   coronary ligaments bind down the outer margins
    of the medial and lateral menisci to the outer
    margins of the tibial condyles.   (   )
b   capsule is pierced posterolaterally by the
    popliteus tendon.   (   )
c   tendinous expansions of the vasti blend with the
    capsule medially and laterally.   (   )
d   tibial collateral ligament is attached to the capsule.   (   )

e   fibular collateral ligament is attached to the apex   (   )
    of the fibula.

229   The synovial membrane of the knee joint:
a   is invaginated from behind by the cruciate ligaments. (   )
b   covers the inferior surface of the menisci.   (   )
c   is continuous with that of the infrapatellar bursa.   (   )
d   is continuous with that of the prepatellar bursa.   (   )
e   surrounds the infrapatellar fold.   (   )

230   The medial meniscus of the knee joint:
a   is formed of fibrocartilage.   (   )

b   is attached to the capsule as well as to the
    condyles of the tibia.   (   )
c   embraces the ends of the lateral meniscus.   (   )

d   gives attachment posteriorly to the tendon of
    popliteus.   (   )
e   gives attachment to the patellar tendon.   (   )

a **T**— It is a synovial joint of the condyloid (modified hinge) variety.
b **F**— The articular cartilage is hyaline.

c **F**— They are in contact in all positions of the joint.

d **F**— The intercondylar ridge completely separates the tibial articular areas and gives attachment to the ends of the
e **T** menisci and both cruciate ligaments.

a **T**— They are capsular thickenings.

b **T**— The tendon has a synovial sheath and is attached to a fossa below the lateral epicondyle.
c **T**— Being known as the patellar retinacula.

d **T**— It has a wide inferior attachment to the medial surface of the tibia. The fibular collateral ligament is separate from the capsule and is attached to the head of the fibula.
e **F**— This is the attachment of biceps; the ligament is attached anterior to this point.

a **T**— These ligaments are intracapsular but extrasynovial.
b **F**— It lines the non-articular surfaces of the joint.
c **F**— The suprapatellar, popliteal and gastrocnemius bursae
d **F** usually communicate with the joint cavity.
e **T**— The fold fans out from the intercondylar notch on the femur to the tibia and lower patella with a 'transverse fringe', the alar fold, on each side.

a **T**— It is wedge-shaped in section and conforms to the adjacent femoral and tibial surfaces.
b **T**— This double attachment makes the medial meniscus less mobile and so more liable to injury.
c **T**— The medial is semicircular, the lateral forms three-fifths of a smaller circle.
d **F**— The tendon is attached to the lateral meniscus which is pulled backwards at the start of the flexion at the knee.
e **F**

231   In movement at the knee joint:

a   flexion is limited by tension in the tibial and fibular
collateral ligaments.   (   )

b   extension is limited by tension in the cruciate,
collateral and oblique popliteal ligaments.   (   )

c   locking of the joint in full extension is by lateral
rotation of the femur on the tibia.   (   )

d   the collateral ligaments limit rotation of the femur
on the tibia.   (   )

e   unlocking of the joint is by medial rotation of the
femur on the tibia by popliteus.   (   )

232   The knee joint:

a   is separated posteriorly from the popliteal vein by
the popliteal artery.   (   )

b   receives an innervation from the obturator nerve.   (   )

c   has an oblique popliteal ligament which is an
extension of the semimembranosus tendon.   (   )

d   lateral femoral condyle is more prominent anteriorly
than the medial.   (   )

e   has the line of weight passing behind the axis of
rolling in the fully extended position.   (   )

233   The superior tibiofibular joint is:

a   a plane synovial joint.   (   )

b   placed on the lateral surface on the lateral tibial
condyle.   (   )

c   medially rotated during dorsiflexion of the ankle.   (   )

d   related anteriorly to the tibialis anterior muscle.   (   )

e   related posteriorly to the tibialis posterior muscle.   (   )

a **F**— The movement is limited by the apposition of the surfaces of the calf and thigh.

b **T**— The attachment of the anterior cruciate ligament fixes the lateral condyle, final extension being accompanied by

c **F** medial rotation of the femur on the tibia. The direction of the fibres in the collateral and oblique posterior ligaments

d **T** is such that it limits this rotation.

e **F**— In unlocking, popliteus laterally rotates the femur on the tibia and also draws the lateral meniscus clear of the condylar surfaces.

a **T**— The tibial nerve is superficial to both vessels.

b **T**— And from the femoral and sciatic nerves which supply the muscles acting on the joint.

c **T**— As is also the fascia over the popliteus muscle.

d **T**— This prominence helps prevent lateral dislocation of the patella during extension at the knee joint.

e **F**— The line passes in front of the axis.

a **T**— The joint cavity may rarely communicate with that of the knee joint. The inferior joint is a fibrous joint.

b **F**— It is situated on the posteroinferior surface of the lateral condyle.

c **F**— Little movement occurs between the tibia and fibula and certainly no rotation.

d **F**— The extensor digitorum longus and peroneus longus muscles are anterior relations. The popliteus tendon and synovial sheath are the main posterior relations.

e **F**— The muscle has a more distal attachment.

234   The popliteal fossa:
a   has the soleus muscle on its floor.   (   )

b   is crossed by the posterior femoral cutaneous nerve. (   )
c   is bordered laterally by the iliotibial tract.   (   )

d   is bordered medially by the gracilis muscle.   (   )

e   has the common peroneal nerve passing through it
laterally.   (   )

235   The tibialis anterior muscle:
a   passes deep to both the superior and inferior
extensor retinacula of the ankle joint.   (   )
b   has attachments to the fibula and the adjacent
interosseous membrane.   (   )

c   crosses the tendon of extensor hallucis longus in
front of the ankle joint.   (   )
d   is attached distally to the medial cuneiform bone.   (   )

e   is crossed by the anterior tibial artery in front of
the ankle joint.   (   )

236   The peroneus brevis muscle:
a   is separated from the lateral malleolus by the
peroneus longus as their tendons pass across the
ankle joint.   (   )
b   is supplied by the deep peroneal nerve.   (   )

c   is bound down to the lateral malleolus by the
superior and inferior peroneal retinacula.   (   )
d   is attached to the medial cuneiform bone.   (   )

e   has tendinous extensions to most metatarsal bones. (   )

a F— The floor is formed by the popliteal surface of the femur, the capsule of the knee joint and the fascia over the popliteus muscle.

b T— The roof is pierced by the small saphenous vein.

c F— The tract lies anterolateral to the knee joint. The biceps tendon forms the lateral border of the fossa.

d F— Semitendinosus and semimembranosus form the medial border.

e T— The sciatic nerve usually divides into its terminal branches in the upper part of the fossa.

a T— The tendon is surrounded by a separate synovial sheath.

b F— It is attached to the hollowed-out upper two-thirds of the lateral surface of the tibia and the adjacent interosseous membrane.

c F— It remains a medial relation to the extensor hallucis throughout its course.

d T— On its medial surface and to the adjacent base of the first metatarsal bone.

e F— The artery lies laterally.

a F— The peroneus brevis tendon lies closer to the bone.

b F— This nerve supplies the muscles of the anterior compartment. The superficial peroneal nerve supplies the peroneal group of muscles.

c T— Enclosed with peroneus longus in a common synovial sheath.

d F— The inferior surface of this bone gives attachment to peroneus longus. The peroneus brevis tendon is attached to the tubercle on the base of the 5th metatarsal.

e F— This describes the attachment of the tibialis posterior muscle.

151

237 The soleus muscle:

a is the most superficial muscle in the calf. ( )

b has the tibial vessels and nerve lying between it and the gastrocnemius muscle. ( )

c is attached superiorly by its medial head to the superior aspect of the medial femoral condyle. ( )

d is attached by the tendo calcaneus to the middle of the posterior surface of the calcaneus. ( )

e is supplied by the common peroneal nerve. ( )

238 The popliteus muscle:

a is attached to the pit below the lateral epicondyle of the femur. ( )

b passes superficial to the tibial nerve. ( )

c has a tendon surrounded by synovial membrane within the knee joint. ( )

d assists in extension at the knee joint. ( )

e is closely related to the popliteal vein. ( )

239 The flexor hallucis longus muscle:

a is attached superiorly to the lower two-thirds of the posterior surface of the tibia. ( )

b becomes tendinous in the mid-calf. ( )

c lies lateral to the tibial vessels and nerve, posterior to the ankle joint. ( )

d is crossed by the tendon of flexor digitorum longus in the sole of the foot. ( )

e is attached to the base of the middle phalanx on the plantar aspect of the hallux and by slips into its distal phalanx. ( )

a F— The gastrocnemius muscle is more superficial for most of the calf.

b F— These structures lie deep to both gastrocnemius and soleus muscles.

c F— The soleus is attached to the upper end of the fibula, the soleal line on the tibia and a tendinous arch between. Gastrocnemius is attached to the femur.

d T— A bursa and a pad of fat separate the tendon from the upper part of the calcaneal surface.

e F— It is supplied by the tibial nerve.

a T— The line of attachment of the capsule of the knee joint passes between the epicondyle and the pit, which is thus intracapsular.

b F— It is deeply placed in the popliteal fossa and is supplied by a branch of the tibial nerve.

c T— The tendon pierces the posterior capsule, a slip passing to the lateral meniscus retracting it in lateral rotation of the femur at the beginning of flexion. The tendon is intracapsular but extrasynovial.

d F— It laterally rotates the femur on the tibia at the beginning of flexion, so 'unlocking' the knee joint.

e F— The popliteal artery lies between the vein and the muscle.

a F— It is attached to this region of the fibula and adjacent interosseous membrane. (The muscle going to the medial side of the foot (FHL) comes from the lateral bone in the leg. The muscle going to the lateral side (FDL) comes from the medial bone.)

b F— The tendon starts behind the lower end of the tibia.

c T— The tendons of flexor digitorum longus and tibialis posterior are medial to the tendon and vessels.

d T— It then passes forwards in the groove between the sesamoid bones in the two heads of the flexor hallucis brevis.

e F— It is attached to the base of the distal phalanx, plantar flexing the great toe and foot, and supporting the medial longitudinal arch.

240   The popliteal artery:
  a enters the popliteal fossa through the adductor hiatus. ( )
  b lies deep on the lower posterior surface of the femur. ( )
  c gives off the peroneal branch in the lower part of the popliteal fossa. ( )
  d is separated from the common peroneal nerve by the popliteal vein. ( )
  e gives a branch to the extensor compartment of the leg. ( )

241   The popliteal vein:
  a lies subcutaneous in the popliteal fossa. ( )
  b lies between the popliteal artery and tibial nerve. ( )
  c has a prominent branch from the superficial veins of the calf. ( )
  d pierces the deep fascia overlying the popliteal fossa. ( )
  e is closely related to the saphenous nerve. ( )

242   The tibial nerve:
  a lies on tibialis posterior in the upper calf. ( )
  b descends through the calf between flexor digitorum longus medially and flexor hallucis longus laterally. ( )
  c innervates both medial and lateral heads of gastrocnemius. ( )
  d innervates the skin over the back of the leg and the lateral border of the foot through its sural branch. ( )
  e gives rise to the medial plantar nerve. ( )

243   The common peroneal nerve:
  a is a branch of the femoral nerve. ( )
  b divides in the substance of peroneus longus. ( )
  c is subcutaneous as it crosses the neck of the fibula. ( )
  d supplies the three peroneal muscles through its superficial peroneal branch. ( )
  e supplies the skin over the medial border of the hallux through the medial dorsal branch of the superficial peroneal. ( )

a T— As a continuation of the femoral artery.

b T— Then crosses the capsule of the knee joint and the fascia over the popliteus muscle.

c F— The peroneal artery is a branch of the posterior tibial artery.

d F— This is the relation of the tibial nerve. The common peroneal nerve lies laterally in the fossa.

e T— The anterior tibial artery passes forwards above the interosseous membrane into this compartment.

a F— It is deep to the deep fascia, the nerve lying superficial to it

b T   and the artery deep.

c T— The short saphenous vein pierces the roof of the fossa.

d F— It follows the main artery through the adductor hiatus and becomes the femoral vein.

e F— The nerve lies on the medial aspect of the knee.

a T— Inferiorly the nerve is related to the capsule of the ankle

b T   joint and ends deep to the flexor retinaculum.

c T— Also plantaris, popliteus, soleus and the deep muscles of the calf.

d T— A branch of the common peroneal nerve (peroneal communicating nerve) joins the sural nerve.

e T— The medial and lateral plantar nerves are the terminal branches.

a F— It is a branch of the sciatic nerve.

b T— Into superficial and deep peroneal nerves.

c T— An important relation as it can be easily damaged in this region.

d F— The peroneus tertius is supplied by the deep peroneal nerve.

e T— Also the second, third and fourth interdigital clefts, the 1st being supplied by the deep peroneal nerve.

244 **The talus:**

a   articulates with the calcaneus at facets on the under surface of its body and head.   (   )

b   receives a slip from the tibialis posterior tendon on the inferior part of its neck.   (   )

c   is grooved by the tendon of flexor hallucis longus between the lateral and medial tubercles on the posterior border.   (   )

d   has an articular facet for the plantar calcaneonavicular ligament on the inferior aspect of the head.   (   )

e   is grooved by the peroneus brevis and longus tendons.   (   )

245 **The calcaneus:**

a   gives attachment to the plantar calcaneonavicular ligament in the sulcus calcanei.   (   )

b   is grooved by the tibialis posterior tendon on the inferior surface of the sustentaculum tali.   (   )

c   articulates with the talus by the articular facet on the upper surface of the sustentaculum tali.   (   )

d   has the long plantar ligament attached to the anterior tubercle on its inferior surface.   (   )

e   is closely related laterally to the peroneus brevis and longus tendons.   (   )

246 **The cuboid bone:**

a   receives a slip from the tibialis posterior tendon on its inferior surface.   (   )

b   gives attachment to the peroneus brevis tendon.   (   )

c   is grooved by the peroneus longus tendon.   (   )

d   articulates superiomedially with the talus.   (   )

e   has a centre of ossification present at birth.   (   )

a **T**— The concave posterior facet articulates with the posterior facet of the calcaneus, and the head and neck articulate with the anterior and middle calcaneal facets inferiorly.

b **F**— The bone has no muscular attachments.

c **T**— The lateral tubercle gives attachment to the posterior talofibular ligament.

d **T**— The ligament is also known as the spring ligament. The head articulates anteriorly with the navicular bone.

e **F**— These tendons groove the lower end of the fibula.

a **F**— A strong interosseous talocalcaneal ligament is attached in the groove which in the articulated skeleton is turned into a narrow tunnel, the sinus tarsi, by a corresponding groove in the talus.

b **F**— The tendon of flexor hallucis longus lies in this groove.

c **T**— The talus also articulates with the anterior and the posterior facets on the calcaneus.

d **F**— The turbercle gives attachment to the short plantar ligament. The long plantar ligament is attached to the under surface of the calcaneus in front of the medial and lateral processes.

e **T**— The tendons are separated from each other by the peroneal tubercle of the bone.

a **T**— The tendon is primarily attached with the plantar calcaneonavicular ligament to the navicular tuberosity but sends slips to all tarsal bones except the talus.

b **F**— The tendon is attached to the adjacent tubercle on the 5th metatarsal.

c **T**— The peroneus longus tendon grooves the inferior surface of the bone.

d **F**— It lies between the calcaneus and the 4th and 5th metatarsals, and articulates medially with the lateral cuneiform and sometimes the navicular bone.

e **T**— As do the talus and calcaneus. Centres appear in the other tarsal bones in the first 3 years of life.

247   The ankle joint:
a   is a synovial joint between the tibia and fibula superiorly and the trochlear surface of the talus inferiorly.   (   )
b   is more stable in plantar flexion.   (   )
c   has a medial (deltoid) ligament attached inferiorly to the neck of the talus.   (   )
d   has a lateral ligament attached inferiorly to the body of the calcaneus.   (   )
e   has the extensor hallucis longus tendon situated anteriorly in between the anterior tibial vessels laterally and the tibialis anterior tendon medially.   (   )

248   The talocalcaneonavicular joint:
a   is a synovial joint of the ball and socket variety.   (   )
b   has hyaline cartilage lining the articular surface of the plantar calcaneonavicular ligament.   (   )
c   is reinforced by the bifurcate ligament laterally.   (   )
d   is reinforced by the deltoid ligament medially.   (   )
e   is reinforced inferiorly by the short plantar ligament.   (   )

249   In movements of the foot:
a   eversion is increased in plantar flexion.   (   )
b   inversion is increased in plantar flexion.   (   )
c   eversion is produced by the tibialis posterior muscle.   (   )
d   inversion is produced by the tibialis anterior and posterior muscles.   (   )
e   eversion is limited by tension in the deltoid ligament.   (   )

a **T**— The trochlear surface is a continuous articular one formed by the superior, medial and lateral facets.

b **F**— The trochlear surface is wider anteriorly and the joint is thus more stable in dorsiflexion.

c **T**— This triangular ligament has a continuous attachment to the navicular, the neck of the talus, the plantar calcaneonavicular ligament, the sustentaculum tali and the body of the talus.

d **T**— It also has horizontally placed anterior and posterior talofibular parts.

e **T**— The deep peroneal nerve and the tendons of extensor digitorum longus and peroneus tertius are respectively placed lateral to the vessels.

a **T**— This joint in combination with the calcaneocuboid is known as the midtarsal joint. Together the two joints are important in inversion and eversion of the foot.

b **T**— The remainder of the distal articular surface is formed by the cavity of the navicular bone and the anterior and middle facets on the upper surface of the calcaneus.

c **T**— And the deltoid ligament medially. The bifurcate ligament
d **T** passes from the upper calcaneus to the adjacent cuboid and navicular bones.

e **F**— The ligament passes from the anterior calcaneal tubercle to the adjacent surface of the cuboid.

a **F**— The movement is greatest in dorsiflexion.
b **T**— The narrower posterior part of the talus allows movement at the ankle joint in addition to movement at the talocalcaneonavicular joint.

c **F**— It is produced by the peroneus brevis and longus muscles.

d **T**— And limited by tension in the peroneal muscles and the interosseous talocalcaneal ligament.

e **T**— And also by tension in the tibialis muscles. It is produced by the peroneal muscles.

250   The arches of the foot:
a   have the effect of concentrating the weight of the
    body on to a small area.   (   )
b   give the foot resilience.   (   )
c   are dependent largely on bony factors.   (   )

d   are not present at birth.   (   )
e   have more prominent plantar than dorsal ligaments. (   )

251   The medial longitudinal arch of the foot:
a   extends from the medial process of the calcaneus
    to the head of the medial three metatarsals.   (   )
b   is supported by the tibialis posterior muscle.   (   )
c   is supported by the tibialis anterior muscle.   (   )
d   is supported by the peroneus longus tendon.   (   )
e   is supported by the long plantar ligament.   (   )

252   The lateral plantar nerve:
a   is the larger terminal branch of the tibial nerve
    beginning beneath the flexor retinaculum.   (   )
b   supplies the flexor accessorius muscle.   (   )

c   innervates the skin of the plantar aspect of the
    lateral three and a half toes.   (   )
d   supplies flexor digitorum brevis.   (   )
e   supplies abductor hallucis.   (   )

253   The deep fascia of the lower limb:
a   is attached superiorly to the sacrotuberous ligament. (   )

b   has the saphenous opening 1 cm below and medial
    to the pubic tubercle.   (   )
c   helps to stabilise the knee through the attachment
    of the lower fibres of the adductor magnus muscle. (   )

d   is thickened laterally at the ankle as the flexor
    retinaculum.   (   )
e   forms the plantar aponeurosis.   (   )

a F— They allow weight to be spread over a larger area.

b T— Which makes it well suited to absorb impacts.

c F— The maintenance of the arches is dependent on muscular, ligamentous and bony factors which are complementary to one another.

d F— They are present though masked by subcutaneous fat.

e T— They are stronger and more numerous.

a T— The talus, navicular and three cuneiform bones also take part.

b T— Tying together the posterior bones of the arch.

c T— Through its attachment near the centre of the arch.

d F— This supports the lateral and transverse arches.

e F— This passes to the base of the 4th and 5th metatarsal bones and supports the lateral longitudinal arch.

a F— The medial plantar nerve is the larger branch but has the smaller distribution.

b T— This muscle contracts when the flexor hallucis longus and flexor digitorum longus are relaxing.

c F— It supplies the lateral one and a half toes.

d F— The flexor digitorum brevis, abductor hallucis, flexor

e F hallucis brevis and the 1st lumbrical are supplied by the medial plantar nerve. The lateral supplies the other short muscles of the sole.

a T— The fascia has a continuous attachment to the pubic bone, inguinal ligament, iliac crest, back of the sacrum, the sacrotuberous ligament and the ischiopubic ramus.

b F— The opening is 3 cm below and 1 cm lateral to the tubercle.

c F— Its thickening in the thigh, the iliotibial tract, receives fibres from the gluteus maximus and tensor fasciae latae muscles and helps to stabilise and extend the knee joint.

d F— The flexor tendons lie medially. The deep fascia is thickened around the ankle joint as the retinacula, and over

e T the sole as the plantar aponeurosis.

254 The great saphenous vein:
  a passes behind the medial malleolus.   (   )
  b passes anterior to the knee joint.   (   )

  c is accompanied by the saphenous nerve in the
     lower leg.   (   )
  d enters the femoral vein in the middle of the thigh.   (   )

  e usually receives blood from the deep veins in the
     legs and thighs.   (   )

255 In the lymph drainage of the lower limb:
  a the deep vessels pass with the limb arteries.   (   )
  b the popliteal nodes receive afferents from the
     area drained by the small saphenous vein.   (   )

  c efferent vessels from the upper superficial inguinal
     group pass to the nodes around the umbilicus.   (   )
  d the deep inguinal nodes lie in the femoral canal.   (   )

  e the gluteal region drains to the pararectal nodes.   (   )

**256 In peripheral nerve injuries of the lower limb; section of
the:**
  a obturator nerve rarely produces loss of cutaneous
     sensation.   (   )
  b tibial nerve produces loss of dorsiflexion and
     eversion of the foot.   (   )
  c deep peroneal nerve gives sensory loss over the
     medial aspect of the foot.   (   )

  d femoral nerve gives sensory loss over the medial
     aspect of the thigh and leg.   (   )
  e femoral nerve produces loss of hip extension.   (   )

a **F**— It is formed at the medial end of the dorsal venous arch and
b **F**   passes anterior to the medial malleolus and then posterior to the knee.
c **T**— The nerve can be damaged in surgery on the vein at this level.

d **F**— The union is in the upper thigh. The great saphenous vein passes through the saphenous opening in the deep fascia and joins the femoral vein.
e **F**— The valvular arrangement in the communicating veins is such as to direct blood from the superficial to the deep systems.

a **T**— The superficial vessels pass with the superficial veins.
b **T**— This is the lateral side of the foot and leg. The nodes lie around the termination of the vein deep to the popliteal fascia.
c **F**— There are no lymph nodes on the anterior abdominal wall. This area drains down to the groin and up to the axilla.
d **T**— They comprise one to three nodes and receive lymph from all superficial nodes and the deep vessels from the entire limb.
e **F**— This region drains to the superficial inguinal nodes.

a **T**— However, adduction is limited to the fibres of adductor magnus innervated by the sciatic nerve.
b **F**— These are the defects produced by damage of the common peroneal nerve.
c **F**— The only cutaneous loss is over the first interdigital cleft. There is loss of dorsiflexion and the foot becomes inverted by the unopposed action of tibialis posterior (foot drop).
d **T**— Due to damage of the medial femoral cutaneous and saphenous nerves.
e **F**— The quadriceps femoris muscle is paralysed, with loss of extension at the knee joint.

163

257   In the normal stance the:

a   centre of gravity lies just anterior to the 2nd
lumbar vertebra.   (   )

b   line of weight passes slightly behind the axis of
the hip joint.   (   )

c   line of weight passes slightly behind the axis of
the knee joint.   (   )

d   weight of the body tends to dorsiflex the body
over the feet.   (   )

e   the digital extensors hold the toes on the ground.   (   )

VIII Head and Neck

258   On the superior aspect of the skull the:

a   sutures are all fibrous joints.   (   )

b   coronal suture separates the frontal from the
parietal bones.   (   )

c   bregma lies between the sagittal and lambdoid
sutures.   (   )

d   anterior fontanelle is usually closed at birth.   (   )

e   posterior fontanelle is usually closed by the
2nd–3rd month after birth.   (   )

259   On the anterior aspect of the skull the:

a   inferior orbital margin is formed by the maxillary
and zygomatic bones.   (   )

•b   infraorbital foramen is situated at approximately
the junction of the middle and lateral thirds of the
inferior orbital margin.   (   )

c   lateral wall of the orbit is formed by the frontal
and zygomatic bones and the greater wing of the
sphenoid.   (   )

d   medial orbital margin is formed by the frontal,
lacrimal and maxillary bones.   (   )

e   nasal aperture is produced by the frontal, nasal,
maxillary and temporal bones.   (   )

a F— It lies just anterior to the second piece of the sacrum.

b T— Hyperextension is limited by tension in the iliofemoral ligament and the contraction of the iliopsoas muscle.

c F— It passes just in front of the axis of the joints, hyperextension being limited by the ligaments and the contraction of the hamstrings and gastrocnemius muscles.

d T— This is resisted by the action of the calf muscles, especially soleus.

e F— This action is brought about by the long digital flexors.

a T— After middle age, the inner aspect of the sutures starts to ossify.

b T— At birth, the two halves of the frontal bone are separated by the frontal suture.

c F— The lambda (posterior fontanelle) is situated in this position. The bregma (anterior fontanelle) is between the sagittal, coronal and frontal sutures.

d F— The anterior fontanelle is diamond-shaped and usually
e T   closed about 18 months after birth.

a T— This can be palpated in its whole length. Medially it ends in the lacrimal fossa.

b F— It lies at the junction of the middle and medial thirds in line with the supraorbital notch and mental foramen.

c T— The frontozygomatic suture can be palpated on the lateral orbital margin in the living.

d F— The lacrimal bone forms part of the medial orbital wall but not its margin.

e F— The frontal and zygomatic bones are not involved.

260 **On the lateral aspect of the skull the:**

a   pterion is sited approximately 3.45 cm behind and 1.5 cm above the frontozygomatic suture.   (   )

b   infratemporal fossa communicates with the pterygopalatine fossa through the pterygotympanic fissure.   (   )

c   zygomatic arch is formed by the zygomatic and sphenoid bones.   (   )

d   external acoustic meatus is formed antero-inferiorly by the tympanic plate of the temporal bone.   (   )

e   mastoid process is partly formed by the occipital bone.   (   )

261 **On the inferior aspect of the skull the:**

a   hard palate is formed by the maxillary, vomer and palatine bones.   (   )

b   incisive.foramen transmits the greater and lesser palatine nerves.   (   )

c   incisive foramen transmits the greater palatine artery. (   )

d   posterior nares (nasal apertures) are formed laterally by the medial pterygoid plates.   (   )

e   pterygoid hamulus gives attachment to the tensor veli palatini muscle.   (   )

262 **On the inferior aspect of the skull the:**

a   foramen ovale transmits the maxillary nerve.   (   )

b   spine of the sphenoid gives attachment to the sphenomandibular ligament.   (   )

c   foramen spinosum transmits the middle meningeal artery.   (   )

d   squamotympanic fissure is continuous medially with the petrosquamous and petrotympanic fissures.   (   )

e   petrotympanic fissure transmits the chorda tympani nerve.   (   )

a **T**— This is the H-shaped union of the frontal, temporal, parietal and sphenoid bones. It overlies the anterior branches of the middle meningeal vessels.

b **F**— The communication is through the pterygomaxillary fissure.

c **F**— The arch is formed by the zygomatic process of the squamous temporal bone and the temporal process of the zygomatic bone.

d **T**— It is completed posterosuperiorly by the squamous temporal bone.

e **F**— It is a part of the temporal bone.

a **F**— The vomer separates the posterior nares but does not form part of the palate. It articulates with the upper surface of the palate.

b **F**— The greater and lesser palatine nerves have their own foramina opening on the posterolateral aspect of the palate.

c **T**— The foramina in the incisive fossa transmit the nasopalatine nerves and the terminal branches of the greater palatine arteries.

d **T**— And superiorly by the body of the sphenoid, medially by the vomer.

e **F**— The tendon of this muscle hooks around the hamulus, but the pterygomandibular raphe and the superior constrictor are attached to it.

a **F**— It transmits the mandibular nerve.

b **T**— Both structures are derived from the cartilage of the first pharyngeal arch.

c **T**— This is a branch of the maxillary artery and supplies both the dura and the skull bones. It can be damaged in skull fractures.

d **T**— A thin projection of the petrous part of the temporal bone subdivides the squamotympanic fissure into these two parts.

e **T**— This nerve carries sensory fibres (especially taste) from the anterior two-thirds of the tongue (lingual nerve) and the secretomotor fibres to the submandibular ganglion.

263 **On the inferior aspect of the skull the:**
a foramen lacerum is pierced by the internal carotid artery. ( )
b medial of the two grooves on the medial aspect of the mastoid process houses the occipital artery. ( )
c tip of the styloid process gives attachment to the stylomandibular ligament. ( )
d the stylomastoid foramen transmits the vestibulocochlear nerve. ( )
e hypoglossal nerve passes through the posterior condylar foramen. ( )

264 **The mandible:**
a gives attachment to the lateral pterygoid muscle along the coronoid process. ( )
b gives attachment to the medial pterygoid muscle along the coronoid process. ( )
c has the lingual nerve crossing the root of the 3rd molar tooth. ( )
d gives attachment to the sphenomandibular ligament at the lingula. ( )
e develops in the cartilage of the first pharyngeal arch (Meckel's cartilage). ( )

265 **The maxilla:**
a has a rounded tuberosity at the posterior aspect of the alveolar process. ( )
b has a large opening on its medial surface. ( )
c has the infraorbital nerve and vessels running through its superior surface. ( )
d contributes to the floor of the orbit. ( )
e develops in cartilage from a centre above the canine tooth. ( )

266 **The sphenoid bone transmits the:**
a mandibular branch of the trigeminal nerve. ( )
b middle meningeal artery. ( )
c internal carotid artery. ( )
d optic nerve. ( )
e ophthalmic nerve. ( )

a **F**— The foramen in life is filled with cartilage which forms the floor of the carotid canal medially.

b **T**— The lateral gives attachment to the posterior belly of the digastric muscle.

c **F**— The stylohyoid ligament is attached at this site. Both ligament and process are derived from the cartilage of the 2nd pharyngeal arch.

d **F**— It transmits the facial nerve.

e **F**— The nerve passes through the anterior (hypoglossal) foramen. The posterior transmits an emissary vein.

a **F**— The muscle is attached to the fossa on the front of the neck of the mandible. The temporalis muscle is attached to the coronoid process.

b **F**— It is attached to the medial surface of the ramus below the mandibular foramen.

c **T**— This is an important landmark in dental anaesthesia.

d **T**— Both are derived from the cartilage of 1st pharyngeal arch.

e **F**— The bone develops in the mesenchyme lateral to this cartilage which later disappears as the bone grows round it.

a **T**— One head of the medial pterygoid muscle is attached here.

b **T**— This is largely covered in the articulated skull by the bones of the lateral wall of the nose, especially the inferior concha.

c **T**— The bone in this region is thin and the nerve is usually damaged in maxillary fractures.

d **T**— The thin superior surface forms the larger part of the orbital floor.

e **F**— It develops in mesenchyme from a centre in this region.

a **T**— Via the foramen ovale in the greater wing.

b **T**— Via the foramen spinosum in the greater wing.

c **F**— The artery rests on the superior surface of the body of the sphenoid.

d **T**— Through the optic canal where it is surrounded by a sheath of the meninges and the subarachnoid space.

e **F**— Branches of the nerve pass into the orbit between the greater and lesser wings of the sphenoid.

267 **The body of the sphenoid:**
a articulates anteriorly with the frontal bone. ( )

b forms the roof of the nasopharynx. ( )

c projects posterosuperiorly as the dorsum sellae. ( )
d forms the inferior relation of the cavernous sinus. ( )
e ossifies in cartilage. ( )

268 **The temporal bone transmits the:**
a trigeminal nerve. ( )

b facial nerve. ( )

c abducent nerve. ( )

d vestibulocochlear nerve. ( )

e glossopharyngeal nerve. ( )

269 **The petrous part of the temporal bone:**
a contains the carotid canal. ( )

b transmits the greater petrosal nerve. ( )

c transmits the lesser petrosal nerve. ( )

d forms the floor of the external acoustic meatus. ( )

e is closely related to the internal jugular vein. ( )

a F— The lesser wings articulate with the orbital plate of the frontal bone on each side and the ethmoid medially.

b T— Small collections of lymphoid tissue in this region form the pharyngeal tonsil (adenoids).

c T— This forms the posterior boundary of the pituitary fossa.

d T— On either side of the pituitary fossa.

e T— Only the pterygoid processes and the lateral part of the greater wings ossify in mesenchyme.

a F— The trigeminal ganglion grooves the apex of the petrous temporal bone.

b T— This nerve enters by the internal acoustic meatus and leaves through the stylomastoid foramen.

c F— This nerve leaves the cranial cavity through the superior orbital fissure having crossed the apex of the petrous temporal bone.

d T— The nerve enters the internal acoustic meatus to reach the inner ear.

e F— It passes through the jugular foramen formed between temporal and occipital bones.

a T— The canal transmits the internal carotid artery surrounded with a plexus of sympathetic nerves.

b T— This nerve leaves the facial nerve at the geniculate ganglion and becomes the nerve of pterygoid canal.

c T— This nerve comes from the tympanic plexus and passes to the otic ganglion.

d F— It contains the internal acoustic meatus which transmits the facial and vestibulocochlear nerves and the labyrinthine vessels.

e T— The jugular foramen is bounded by the temporal and occipital bones.

270   **The styloid process:**
  a   gives attachment to the styloglossus muscle
      near its tip.   (   )
  b   gives attachment to a muscle supplied by the
      glossopharyngeal nerve.   (   )
  c   gives attachment to a muscle supplied by the
      facial nerve.   (   )
  d   gives attachment to a muscle supplied by the
      vagus nerve.   (   )
  e   ossifies in cartilage.   (   )

271   **The occipital bone:**
  a   gives attachment to the oblique capitis inferior
      muscle.   (   )

  b   is grooved by the superior sagittal sinus.   (.)

  c   transmits the vestibulocochlear nerve.   (   )

  d   transmits the vagus nerve.   (   )

  e   develops mostly in cartilage.   (   )

272   **The frontal bone:**
  a   transmits the zygomatic nerve.   (   )

  b   articulates with the greater wing of the sphenoid.   (   )
  c   articulates with the zygomatic bones.   (   )
  d   gives attachment to the temporalis muscle.   (   )
  e   articulates only with bones formed in mesenchyme.   (   )

a **T**— This is the lowest of its three muscle attachments. The muscle is supplied by the hypoglossal nerve.

b **T**— Stylopharyngeus is the only muscle supplied by this nerve.

c **T**— The stylohyoid muscle. It is attached between the other two styloid muscles.

d **F**

e **T**— From the cartilage of the 2nd pharyngeal arch which also gives rise to the stapes and part of the hyoid bone. The squamous and tympanic parts of the temporal bone ossify in mesenchyme. The petromastoid part of the temporal bone ossifies in cartilage (part of the chondrocranium). The malleus and incus arise from the 1st pharyngeal arch cartilage.

a **F**— This muscle passes from the spine of the axis to the transverse mass of the atlas. The superior oblique is attached to the occiput.

b **T**— This is usually in continuity with the right transverse venous sinus.

c **F**— This passes into the internal acoustic meatus of the petrous temporal bone. The hypoglossal nerve emerges through a foramen in front of the occipital condyle.

d **F**— The bone borders the jugular foramen that transmits the nerve.

e **T**— Only the squamous portion (above the superior nuchal line) develops in mesenchyme.

a **F**— The facial and temporal branches of this nerve pass through small foramina in the zygomatic bone.

b **T**— In the lateral wall of the orbit.

c **T**— Along the lateral orbital margin.

d **T**— In the temporal fossa.

e **F**— The ethmoid and the lesser wings of the sphenoid bones are the exceptions.

273 **The ethmoid bone:**
  a forms part of the medial wall of the orbit. (   )

  b forms the inferior conchae. (   )

  c articulates with the nasal bone. (   )
  d articulates with the vomer. (   )

  e is perforated by the olfactory nerves. (   )

274 **The palatine bone:**
  a has a tubercle which separates the maxilla from the pterygoid process of the sphenoid bone. (   )
  b forms part of the roof of the mouth. (   )

  c articulates with the medial pterygoid plate. (   )

  d meets the maxilla and forms the nasolacrimal duct. (   )

  e forms part of the nasal septum. (   )

275 **The hyoid bone:**
  a gives attachment of the superior constrictor muscles. (   )

  b is attached by a muscle to the scapula. (   )
  c gives attachment to a muscle supplied by the facial nerve. (
  d gives attachment to a muscle supplied by the hypoglossal nerve. (
  e is mainly derived from the 4th pharyngeal arch cartilage. (

276 **The scalp:**
  a is attached by the occipitalis muscle to the skull. (
  b is attached by the frontalis muscle to the skull. (
  c receives sensory innervation from the dorsal rami of the 2nd and 3rd cervical nerves. (
  d receives part of its blood supply from the ophthalmic artery. (
  e drains directly to the deep lymph nodes around the carotid sheath. (

a **T**— The ethmoidal labyrinth lies between the orbit and the nasal cavity.

b **F**— This is a separate bone but the superior and middle conchae are part of the ethmoid.

c **F**— The nasal process of the frontal bone lies between them.

d **T**— By its perpendicular plate. Together they form the bony portions of the nasal septum.

e **T**— Through the cribriform plate.

a **T**

b **T**— It lies between the palatine part of the maxilla and the soft palate.

c **T**— With it forming the posterior aspect of the lateral wall of the nose.

d **F**— The bone does meet the maxilla but the greater palatine canal is formed.

e **T**— With its vertical plate.

a **F**— The middle constrictor is attached to the greater and lesser horns and the stylohyoid ligament.

b **T**— By the omohyoid muscle.

c **T**— Both the stylohyoid and the posterior belly of digastric are supplied by the facial nerve.

d **T**— Hyoglossus is attached to the body and greater horn of the hyoid bone.

e **F**— It develops from the cartilages of the 2nd and 3rd arches.

a **T**— The muscle is attached to the superior nuchal line.

b **F**— The frontalis is not attached to bone.

c **T**— Via the greater and 3rd occipital nerves behind the vertex. The trigeminal nerve supplies in front of the vertex.

d **T**— Via the supraorbital and supratrochlear branches of the ophthalmic artery.

e **F**— A superficial circle of lymph nodes around the lower parts of the skull first receives the lymph drained from the scalp.

277 **The facial muscles:**
   a are embedded in the deep fascia of the face.   ( )

   b are derived from the mesenchyme of the second
       pharyngeal arch.   ( )
   c share a common raphe with a constrictor muscle. ( )

   d gain a bony attachment through the medial
       palpebral ligament.   ( )
   e have no bony attachments.   ( )

278 **Buccinator:**
   a is attached to both maxilla and mandible.   ( )
   b blends with orbicularis oculi.   ( )

   c has vertical muscle fibres.   ( )
   d is used during chewing.   ( )
   e is supplied by the trigeminal nerve.   ( )

279 **In the development of the face the:**
   a mandibular process is derived from the 2nd
       pharyngeal arch.   ( )
   b maxillary process is developed from the 1st
       pharyngeal arch.   ( )
   c greater palatine canal develops along the line of
       fusion of the frontonasal and maxillary processes. ( )
   d part of the upper jaw bearing the incisor teeth
       develops from the frontonasal process.   ( )
   e the forehead is formed from the maxillary
       processes.   ( )

280 **The superior orbital fissure:**
   a is bounded by the greater wing of the sphenoid
       and the orbital plate of the frontal bone.   ( )
   b links the orbit with the pterygopalatine fossa. ( )

   c transmits the optic nerve.   ( )

   d transmits the trochlear nerve within the common
       tendinous ring of attachment of the extraocular
       muscles.   ( )
   e transmits the lacrimal nerve within the common
       tendinous ring.   ( )

a F— There is no deep fascia on the face, other than that over the parotid gland.

b T— They are supplied by the nerve of the arch, the facial nerve.

c T— The pterygomandibular raphe unites the buccinator and superior constrictor muscles.

d T— This ligament receives fibres from the orbicularis oculi and is attached to the frontal process of the maxilla.

e F— Ocular muscles are attached to bone medially, and oral to the zygoma and mandible.

a T— It is attached to both bones and the pterygomandibular
b F   raphe and its transverse fibres pass forwards to blend with those of orbicularis oris.

c F

d T— Its action helps to keep food between the teeth in chewing.

e F— It is supplied by the facial nerve.

a F— The mandibular process is a derivative of the 1st
b T   pharyngeal arch and the maxillary process also grows from the mandibular process.

c F— The nasolacrimal duct is formed along this line of fusion.

d T— This premaxillary portion is formed from the median nasal process of the frontonasal process.

e F— It is formed from the frontonasal process.

a F— It lies between the greater and lesser wings of the sphenoid, linking the orbit with the middle cranial fossa.

b F— This fossa communicates with the orbit through the inferior orbital fissure.

c F— The nerve enters the orbit through the optic canal between the body and the lesser wing of sphenoid.

d F— The lacrimal, frontal and trochlear nerves pass through the fissure outside this attachment. The nasociliary, oculomotor and abducent nerves are within the ring.

e F

281 In the eyeball:

a the cornea is a derivative of the choroid layer. (   )

b the fovea centralis represents the site of entry of the optic nerve into the eyeball. (   )

c the posterior chamber of the eye is filled with vitreous substance. (   )

d ciliary muscle contraction produces a more convex lens. (   )

e the medial check ligament is attached to the maxillary bone. (   )

282 In the eyeball the:

a ciliary branches of the ophthalmic artery supply the macular area. (   )

b long ciliary nerves come from the ciliary ganglion and pierce the sclera posteriorly. (   )

c iris is developed from the mesenchyme. (   )

d medial check ligament is attached to the frontal process of the maxillary bone. (   )

e suspensory ligament is an extension of the superior oblique tendon. (   )

283 In movements of the eyeball:

a downward and medial movement is initiated through the inferior division of the oculomotor nerve. (   )

b lateral movement is mediated through the superior division of the oculomotor nerve. (   )

c upward and medial movement is mediated through the abducent nerve. (   )

d downward and lateral movement is initiated through the trochlear nerve. (   )

e medial movement is mediated through the abducent nerve. (   )

a F— The cornea is derived as a condensation of the mesenchyme over the optic cup.
b F— The fovea and the macula lie lateral to the nerve entry and are used mainly for daylight vision.
c F— This chamber lies between the lens and the iris, and is filled with aqueous humor.
d T— The circular ciliary muscle is supplied by the parasympathetic fibres in the oculomotor nerve. The increased convexity is produced by the inherent elasticity of the lens when the suspensory ligament (zonular fibres) is relaxed.
e F— The medial and lateral check ligaments are respectively attached to the lacrimal and zygomatic bones.

a F— The central artery of the retina, a branch of the ophthalmic artery, supplies the macula and the rest of the retina.
b F— These nerves are branches of the nasociliary nerve and are sensory to the cornea. The ganglion gives rise to the short ciliary nerves which contain the postganglionic parasympathetic (constrictor) fibres to the ciliary body and iris.
c F— Like the optic nerve and retina, it is a derivative of the primitive forebrain and hence of ectoderm.
d F— It, like the lateral check and suspensory ligaments, is a thickening of the orbital fascia. It is attached to the lacrimal bone.
e F— It is a thickening of the orbital fascia.

a T— The muscle being the inferior rectus.

b F— The lateral rectus is supplied by the abducent nerve.

c F— The superior rectus muscle is supplied by the superior division of the oculomotor nerve.
d T— The muscle being the superior oblique.

F— The medial rectus is supplied by the inferior division of the oculomotor nerve.

284 **The ophthalmic artery:**
a   arises from the internal carotid artery soon after it
     pierces the dura and enters the subarachnoid space. (   )

b   enters the orbit through the superior orbital fissure. (   )
c   passes from medial to lateral over the optic nerve as
     these structures pass anteriorly through the orbit. (   )

d   terminates by dividing into supraorbital and
     infratrochlear branches. (   )
e   supplies the eyeball through the central branch of the
     supratrochlear artery. (   )

285 **In the eyelid the:**
a   tarsal plate is formed of elastic cartilage. (   )
b   tarsal glands are modified sweat glands. (   )
c   tarsal plate is attached to the medial palpebral
     ligament. (   )
d   posterior lining is ciliated columnar epithelium. (.)

e   conjunctival fornix is lined by ciliated columnar
     epithelium. (

286 **In the lacrimal apparatus:**
a   the lacrimal gland is innervated by the
     zygomaticotemporal nerve. (

b   the gland is superficial to the orbicularis oculi
     muscle. (

c   removal of tears is entirely by evaporation from the
     exposed surface of the eyeball. (

d   the nasolacrimal duct descends between the
     maxillary bone and the inferior concha. (
e   the lacrimal canaliculi are lined by stratified
     squamous epithelium. (

a **T**— The internal carotid artery also gives off pituitary, trigeminal, posterior communicating and anterior choroidal branches before dividing into the anterior and the middle cerebral arteries.

b **F**— It traverses the optic canal with the optic nerve.

c **F**— The artery passes from lateral to medial over the optic nerve in company with the nasociliary nerve and near to the ciliary ganglion.

d **F**— The usual termination is into the supratrochlear and dorsal nasal arteries.

e **F**— The central artery of the retina is a direct branch of the ophthalmic.

a **F**— It is formed of firm fibrous tissue.

b **F**— These are modified sebaceous glands.

c **T**— Also to the lateral palpebral ligament.

d **F**— The conjunctiva has mainly a thin layer of stratified columnar epithelium. Over the cornea it is stratified

e **F** squamous and firmly adherent.

a **T**— From the superior salivary nucleus fibres run with the facial nerve and its greater petrosal branch to the pterygopalatine ganglion. Postganglionic fibres run in the zygomaticotemporal branch of the maxillary nerve to the lacrimal branch of the ophthalmic nerve.

b **F**— Much of the gland is surrounded by fibres of orbicularis oculi which help in the expulsion of the tears from the gland.

c **F**— Evaporation may occur under normal conditions but when excessive tears (e.g. in crying) are produced, the extra fluid passes from the lacrimal puncta into the canaliculi (about 10 mm long), under the medial palpebral ligament and into the lacrimal sac.

d **T**— It opens on to the inferior meatus of the nose.

e **T**— The lacrimal sac is lined by stratified columnar epithelium and the nasolacrimal duct by columnar epithelium that is ciliated in places.

287 **The nasal cavity is:**
a partly roofed by the cribriform plate of the ethmoid bone. ( )
b partly floored by the inferior concha. ( )
c limited medially by the ethmoid bone. ( )

d limited laterally by the ethmoid and the palatine bones. ( )

e innervated medially by the anterior ethmoidal nerve. ( )

288 **On the lateral wall of the nose:**
a the sphenoidal air sinus opens into the spheno-ethmoidal recess. ( )
b the bulla ethmoidalis is sited under the middle concha. ( )
c the maxillary air sinus opens in the hiatus semilunaris. ( )
d the frontonasal duct of the frontal air sinus opens into the hiatus semilunaris. ( )

e the inferior meatus has no openings on its lateral wall. ( )

289 **The lateral wall of the nose:**
a has the lacrimal sac lying between the lacrimal and maxillary bones. ( )
b is partly lined by pseudostratified ciliated columnar epithelium with goblet cells. ( )

c anteriorly, drains to the parotid lymph nodes. ( )

d has an upper posterior quadrant supplied by the nasal branches of the maxillary nerve. ( )
e has a lower anterior quadrant supplied by the olfactory nerves. ( )

a T— Also the body of the sphenoid, the nasal and frontal bones, and the nasal cartilages.

b F— The maxilla and palatine bones form the floor.

c T— The vertical plate of this bone together with the vomer and the septal cartilages form the medial wall.

d T— The inferior concha overlies the large defect in the medial surface of the maxilla. The medial pterygoid plate is found posteriorly.

e T— Also the nasopalatine nerve.

a T— The recess is above the superior concha.

b T— The bulla is formed by ethmoidal air cells which open on its surface.

c F— The hiatus is a groove below the bulla ethmoidalis; near its middle is the opening of the maxillary sinus.

d T— The opening is anterosuperior to that of the maxillary sinus, so that the frontal sinus tends to drain into the maxillary sinus.

e F— The nasolacrimal duct opens anteriorly. Behind the meatus, on the pharyngeal wall, is the opening of the auditory tube.

a T— The sac is thin-walled and lies near the skin at the inner angle of the orbit.

b T— This respiratory-type epithelium covers most of the wall, the upper part being lined by olfactory mucosa. The whole region is very vascular.

c F— This region drains to the submandibular nodes, and the posterior part to the retropharyngeal nodes.

d T— The anterior superior, alveolar, and greater palatine branches of the maxillary, and the anterior ethmoidal

e F branch of the ophthalmic nerves contribute to the remainder of the lateral wall. The arteries generally correspond. Olfactory mucosa is limited to the roof and upper part of the septum and lateral wall.

290   The maxillary air sinus:
a   projects laterally into the zygomatic bone.   (   )
b   is grooved by the anterior ethmoidal nerve.   (   )

c   is related to the upper teeth except the incisors.   (   )

d   has a small opening high on its medial wall.   (   )
e   is partly formed medially by the sphenoid bone.   (   )

291   In the oral cavity the:
a   posterior limit is at the level of the palatopharyngeus
    muscle in the posterior arch (pillar) of the fauces.   (   )
b   parotid duct opens opposite the crowns of the
    second premolar tooth.   (   )
c   upper incisors have a bilateral innervation from the
    anterior superior alveolar nerves.   (   )
d   submandibular duct opens at the root of the second
    lower premolar tooth.   (   )
e   the frenulum passes from the tongue to the base of
    the anterior arch of the fauces.   (   )

292   In the gingivae (gums) the:
a   upper labial surface is partly supplied by the
    zygomatic nerve.   (   )
b   upper lingual surface is partly supplied by the
    anterior ethmoidal nerve.   (   )
c   lower labial surface is partly supplied by the facial
    nerve.   (   )
d   lower lingual surface is partly supplied by the inferior
    alveolar nerve.   (   )
e   mucous membrane is of the stratified squamous
    variety.   (

a F— But it does extend into the zygomatic process of the maxilla.

b F— The posterior superior alveolar nerve grooves its posterior wall. The inferior orbital nerve grooves its upper surface, passing into the infraorbital canal anteriorly.

c T— Although the premaxilla develops from the frontonasal process it is incorporated into the maxillary bone. The roots of the premolar and molar teeth, with a thin bony covering, often project into the sinus but the incisors (on the premaxilla) are not related.

d T— Drainage being, therefore, poor.

e F— The medial wall is overlapped by the inferior concha, and to a lesser extent by the lacrimal, ethmoid and palatine bones.

a F— The anterior arch (pillar) of the fauces formed by the palatoglossus muscle is the posterior limit of the cavity.

b F— It opens opposite the crown of the upper 2nd molar tooth.

c T— These branches of the infraorbital nerve are formed in the infraorbital canal.

d F— It opens on the floor of the mouth near the midline on each side of the frenulum of the tongue.

e F— It passes in the midline from the tongue to the floor of the mouth.

a F— The infraorbital and posterior superior alveolar nerves supply this region.

b F— It is innervated by the nasopalatine and greater palatine nerves.

c F— It is supplied by the buccal and mental nerves.

d F— This area is supplied by the lingual nerve.

e T— It is vascular and firmly attached to the alveolar margins.

293   The deciduous teeth:
a   start erupting in the 4th month after birth.   (   )

b   are 20 in number.   (   )
c   have only one upper premolar.   (   )
d   are replaced earlier in the upper jaw by permanent
      teeth.   (   )
e   derive their dentine from mesenchyme.   .   (   )

294   In the hard palate:
a   the vomer forms the posterior bony edge.   (   )

b   the incisive foramen transmits the lesser palatine
      artery.   (   )

c   the mucoperiosteum is rich in mucous glands.   (   )
d   the nasopalatine nerve innervates the muco-
      periosteum adjacent to the premolar teeth in the
      adult.   (   )
e   development is mainly by the palatine process of the
      mandibular process on each side.   (   )

295   The soft palate:
a   has different forms of epithelium on its upper and
      lower surfaces.   (   )

b   has an aponeurosis formed from the expanded
      tendons of the levator veli palatini muscles.   (   )
c   gives attachment to the palatoglossus muscle.   (   )
d   possesses muscles mainly innervated by nerve fibres
      arising in the nucleus ambiguus.   (   )

e   receives a sensory innervation from the mandibular
      branch of the trigeminal nerve.   (   )

186

a **F**— The first lower incisor erupts at about 6 months. The first permanent teeth (the first lower molars) appear at about 6 years.

b **T**— I2, C1, M2 — in each half jaw.

c **F**— There are no deciduous premolar teeth.

d **F**— The lower permanent teeth appear slightly earlier.

e **T**— The ectodermal folds growing in from the mouth cavity produce the primary dental lamina. The enamel is derived only from ectoderm. The rest of the tooth is derived from the ectodermal cup and its contained mesenchyme.

a **F**— It is formed from the palatine process of the maxilla and the horizontal plate of the palatine bones.

b **F**— The terminal branch of the greater palatine artery transverses the foramen along with the nasopalatine nerves.

c **T**— They contribute to the unevenness of the oral surface.

d **F**— The nerve traverses the incisive foramen and innervates the area behind the incisor teeth.

e **F**— The palatine process develops from the maxillary process, the palate being completed anteriorly in the midline by the premaxillary process on the frontonasal process, and posteriorly by the horizontal process of the palatine bone.

a **T**— Respiratory pseudostratified ciliated columnar epithelium covers the upper and stratified squamous epithelium the lower surface.

b **F**— The tensor veli palatini tendons from the aponeurosis.

c **T**— The muscle passes into the side of the tongue.

d **T**— The vagus innervates all muscles of the palate except tensor veli palatini through the pharyngeal plexus. The exception is supplied by the medial pterygoid branch of the mandibular nerve.

e **F**— The sensory innervation is from the palatine branches of the maxillary and the glossopharyngeal nerves.

296 **The tongue:**

a has a foramen caecum situated at the base of the frenulum. ( )

b is separated from the epiglottis by the valleculae on each side of the midline. ( )

c has 7–12 circumvallate papillae situated just behind the sulcus terminalis. ( )

d is attached to the hyoid bone by the genioglossus muscle. ( )

e musculature is derived from 2nd pharyngeal arch mesoderm. ( )

297 **The hyoglossus muscle:**

a lies lateral to the styloglossus. ( )

b has a different nerve supply from palatoglossus. ( )

c has the hypoglossal nerve on its lateral surface. ( )

d has the submandibular duct on its medial surface. ( )

e has the submandibular gland wrapped around its posterior border. ( )

298 **On the tongue the:**

a circumvallate papillae are innervated by the glossopharyngeal nerve. ( )

b lymph drainage of the posterior third is to the submandibular lymph nodes. ( )

c lymph drainage of the anterior two-thirds is to the submandibular nodes. ( )

d posterior third develops from two lateral lingual swellings. ( )

e taste impulses from the posterior third travel in the glossopharyngeal nerves and are relayed in the nucleus of the tractus solitarius. ( )

a F— The foramen caecum lies at the apex of the sulcus terminalis on the dorsum of the tongue towards the back.

b T— These are two shallow fossae separated by the midline glossoepiglottic fold.

c F— The papillae lie just in front of the sulcus.

d F— This muscle attaches it to the mental spine of the mandible. Hyoglossus and other muscles help anchor the tongue to the hyoid bone.

e F— It is from suboccipital somites migrating forward and carrying their nerve supply (hypoglossal) with them.

a F— The styloglossus lies laterally. The stylopharynceus is a superolateral relation of hyoglossus muscle.

b T— All the intrinsic and extrinsic muscles except palatoglossus are supplied by the hypoglossal nerve. Palatoglossus is supplied by the nucleus ambiguus through the pharyngeal plexus.

c T— And the lingual artery on its medial surface.

d F— The duct is crossed twice by the lingual nerve on the lateral surface of the muscle.

e F— The gland lies on the lateral surface of the muscle.

a T— Although they lie in front of the sulcus terminalis and this approximates to the divison of the lingual and glossopharyngeal areas of innervation.

b F— The posterior third drains to the retropharyngeal nodes. The tip drains bilaterally to submental nodes and the sides

c T ipsilaterally to the submandibular nodes.

d F— These swellings develop into the anterior two-thirds of the tongue. The posterior third comes from the copula over the 3rd and 4th arches. The muscles are derived from occipital myotomes which migrate ventrally and carry the hypoglossal nerves with them.

e T— As are those of the anterior part which are carried in the lingual and chorda tympani nerves.

299   The digastric muscle:

a   receives an innervation from the hypoglossal nerve. (   )

b   crosses the tip of the transverse process of the atlas. (   )

c   passes between the internal and external carotid
arteries.   (   )

d   has the occipital artery passing along the lower
border of its posterior belly.   (   )

e   is attached to the lateral aspect of the mastoid
process.   (   )

300   The parotid gland:

a   is separated from the submandibular gland by the
sphenomandibular ligament.   (   )

b   is related anteriorly to the lateral pterygoid muscle. (   )

c   is related posteriorly to the sternocleidomastoid
muscle.   (   )

d   has the external carotid artery running superficial to
the facial nerve within its substance.   (   )

e   receives secretomotor fibres from the facial nerve.   (   )

301   The submandibular gland:

a   like the sublingual receives its parasympathetic
innervation from the facial nerve.   (   )

b   is grooved superiorly by the loop of the lingual
artery.   (   )

c   overlies the glossopharyngeal nerve.   (   )

d   is a mixed salivary gland.   (   )

e   develops from second pharyngeal arch mesoderm.   (   )

a **F**— The anterior belly is supplied by the mylohyoid branch of the inferior alveolar nerve and the posterior by the facial nerve.

b **T**— Along with the spinal accessory nerve and other structures.

c **F**— It passes superficial to both arteries.

d **T**— And the posterior auricular artery passes along the upper border of this belly.

e **F**— The posterior belly is attached to a groove on the medial aspect of the mastoid process and the anterior belly to the digastric fossa on the mandible.

a **F**— They are separated by the stylomandibular ligament which is a thickening of the deep fascia, and forms part of the parotid capsule.

b **F**— The anterior surface overlaps the medial pterygoid and masseter muscles and the intervening ramus of the mandible.

c **T**— Also the posterior belly of the digastric muscle and the mastoid process.

d **F**— The nerve is superficial to the artery.

e **F**— The secretomotor (parasympathetic) fibres are from the glossopharyngeal nerve via the otic ganglion and auriculotemporal nerve.

a **T**— Fibres pass in the chorda tympani and lingual nerves, and relay in the submandibular ganglion.

b **F**— The loop of the lingual artery lies posterior to the gland on the middle constrictor. The facial artery passes over the superior surface of the gland.

c **F**— It is related to the hyoglossal nerve on the hyoglossus muscle.

d **T**— Like the sublingual, but not the parotid which is a serous gland.

e **F**— It develops as a tubular endodermal outgrowth from the floor of the mouth.

302 **The submandibular duct:**
  a   lies deep to mylohyoid.   (   )
  b   opens at the base of the frenulum.   (   )

  c   passes deep to the lingual nerve.   (   )
  d   passes superficial to the lingual nerve.   (   )
  e   receives all the sublingual gland secretion.   (   )

303 **The temporomandibular joint:**
  a   lateral ligament is taut when the jaw is elevated. –   (   )

  b   is a condyloid joint.   (   )

  c   has the tendon of the medial pterygoid muscle
      attached to the fibrocartilaginous disc.   (   )

  d   has the chorda tympani nerve as a posterior relation. (   )
  e   is related to the auriculotemporal nerve posteriorly. (   )

304 **The medial pterygoid muscle:**
  a   is attached to the lateral pterygoid plate of the
      sphenoid bone.   (   )
  b   is attached to the maxillary tuberosity.   (   )

  c   is attached to the infratemporal surface of the
      greater wing of the sphenoid.   (   )
  d   is innervated by the buccal nerve.   (   )

  e   together with the lateral pterygoid elevates the
      mandible.   (   )

a T— The duct passes forward from the deep part of the gland
b T   between mylohyoid and hyoglossus to open in the floor of
        the mouth at the sublingual papilla at the base of the
        frenulum.
c T— It is crossed laterally by the lingual nerve which then turns
d T   medial to it.
e F— The sublingual gland partly secretes into the
        submandibular duct but also has 15–20 small ducts
        opening on to the sublingual fold on the floor of the
        mouth.

a T— This is the most stable position of the joint, the condyle
        also being housed in the articular fossa.
b T— It is a synovial joint of the condyloid (modified hinge)
        variety.
c F— The lateral pterygoid muscle is attached to the anterior
        edge of the disc, to the joint capsule and to the neck of the
        mandible.
d T— As the nerve passes through the petrotympanic fissure.
e T   The capsule of the joint is attached to the anterior edge of
        the fissure.

a T— The deep head of the muscle is attached to the medial
        surface of the plate.
b T— By the superficial head. The two heads embrace the lower
        fibres of the lateral pterygoid muscle.
c F— This is the attachment of the upper head of the lateral
        pterygoid muscle.
d F— This is a sensory branch of the mandibular nerve; the
        motor branches of the mandibular nerve supply all the
        muscles of mastication.
e F— The medial elevates and the lateral protrudes and
        depresses the mandible. The axis of rotation is through the
        lingula.

305 The pharynx:
a extends from the base of the skull to the 4th cervical vertebra. ( )

b is supported superiorly by the pharyngobasilar fascia. ( )

c is related posteriorly to the prevertebral fascia. ( )
d is related anteriorly to the pretracheal fascia. ( )

e has a muscular attachment to the pterygomandibular raphe. ( )

306 The middle constrictor muscle:
a lies medial to the superior constrictor. ( )

b is attached anteriorly to the stylomandibular ligament. ( )
c is attached anteriorly to the stylohyoid ligament. ( )
d has the superior laryngeal artery between it and the inferior constrictor. ( )
e is innervated by the glossopharyngeal nerve. ( )

307 The interior of the pharynx:
a is ridged by the salpingopharyngeus muscle. ( )

b receives a sensory innervation from the mandibular nerve. ( )

c receives a sensory innervation from the accessory nerve. ( )
d has the palatine tonsil in the lateral wall. ( )

e has an anterior extension on each side of the larynx known as the vallecula. ( )

a **F**— The latter is the level of the hyoid bone. The oesophagus and trachea commence at the level of the cricoid cartilage, opposite the 6th cervical vertebra.

b **T**— The fascia is the thickened submucosa between the upper border of the superior constrictor muscles and the base of the skull.

c **T**— This covers the prevertebral muscles.

d **F**— The pharynx is related anteriorly to the nose, mouth and larynx, these dividing it into its respective portions.

e **T**— This is the anterior attachment of the superior constrictor muscle.

a **F**— It lies medial to the inferior but lateral to the superior constrictor muscle.

b **F**— It is attached to the lesser and greater horns of the hyoid and the stylohyoid ligament.

c **T**

d **T**— The artery runs with the internal laryngeal nerve.

e **F**— This nerve supplies stylopharyngeus, but all other pharyngeal muscles are supplied by the vagus through the pharyngeal plexus and the nucleus ambiguus.

T— A small diverticulum, the pharyngeal recess, is formed behind it.

F— The pharyngeal branches of the maxillary, glossopharyngeal and vagus nerves provide sensory innervation.

F

T— This lies between the folds of mucous membrane over the palatoglossus and palatopharyngeus muscles.

F— The extension is the piriform fossa.

308 **The palatine tonsil:**

a lies on the middle constrictor muscle. ( )

b is a posterior relation of the palatopharyngeal muscle. ( )

c has its lymph drainage to the submandibular nodes. ( )

d has a sensory innervation from the vagus. ( )

e is a derivative of the first pharyngeal pouch. ( )

309 **The auditory tube:**

a extends laterally into the squamous temporal bone. ( )

b opens medially into the lateral wall of the nose. ( )

c gives attachment to the tensor veli palatini muscle. ( )

d sends lymph vessels to the submandibular lymph nodes. (

e is lined by ciliated columnar epithelium. (

310 **In the development of the pharyngeal arches the:**

a nerve of the 4th arch is the superior laryngeal. (

b external acoustic meatus is derived from the 2nd pharyngeal cleft. (

c sphenomandibular ligament is a remnant of the 2nd pharyngeal arch cartilage. (

d greater and lesser horns of the hyoid bone have the same origin. (

e larynx is derived from cartilage of the 4th and 6th arches. (

a **F**— The superior constrictor separates it from the facial artery and carotid sheath.

b **F**— This muscle lies in the palatopharyngeal arch and is posterior to the tonsil.

c **F**— The primary drainage is to the deep cervical lymph nodes, particularly to the jugulodigastric node.

d **F**— The sensory innervation is from the glossopharyngeal with a small contribution from the lesser palatine nerve.

e **F**— The tonsil is a derivative of the 2nd pouch, the first contributing to the auditory tube, middle ear and mastoid antrum.

a **F**— Its lateral third lies within the petrous temporal bone.

b **F**— The medial opening is in the lateral wall of the nasopharynx.

c **T**— Also the levator veli palatini and salpingopharyngeus muscles. These muscles help to open the tube in swallowing.

d **F**— It drains to the retropharyngeal nodes.

e **T**— With many mucous glands.

a **T**— The recurrent laryngeal nerve supplies the 6th arch.

b **F**— The meatus is derived from the 1st cleft.

c **F**— The 1st arch cartilage is represented by this ligament, Meckel's cartilage, the malleus and the incus. The mandibular division of the trigeminal is the nerve of the 1st arch.

d **F**— The greater horn and lower part of the body are derived from 3rd arch cartilage, the nerve of which is the

e **T** glossopharyngeal. The remainder of the hyoid bone, the stylohyoid ligament, the styloid process and the stapes are 2nd arch derivatives, their nerve being the facial.

311 **The second stage (pharyngeal phase) of swallowing is:**
  a voluntary.
  b initiated through the glossopharyngeal nerve. ( )

  c partly effected through the hypoglossal nerve. ( )
  d partly effected through the maxillary nerve. ( )

  e partly effected through the recurrent laryngeal nerve. ( )

312 **The larynx:**
  a is related anteriorly to the thyroid isthmus. ( )

  b is related laterally to the carotid sheath. ( )
  c is formed partly of yellow elastic cartilage. ( )

  d lies opposite the 3rd–6th cervical vertebrae. ( )
  e gives attachment to muscles supplied by the first
     cervical nerve root. ( )

313 **The thyroid cartilage is united to the cricoid cartilage by:**
  a a pair of secondary cartilaginous joints. ( )
  b the vocal ligaments. ( )
  c the conus elasticus. ( )
  d muscles supplied by the external laryngeal nerve. ( )
  e muscles supplied by the internal laryngeal nerve. ( )

314 **The arytenoid cartilage:**
  a is united to the cricoid by a plane, synovial joint. ( )

  b gives attachment to the vocal ligament. ( )

  c gives attachment to the vestibular ligament. ( )

  d has a muscular process which gives attachment to
     the oblique arytenoid muscle. ( )

  e is covered posteriorly by mucous membrane. ( )

a **F**— Is largely involuntary.

b **T**— Through stimulation of the anterior arch of the fauces. It may also be initiated by stimulation of the soft palate, oropharynx and epiglottis.

c **F**— The tongue is closely involved in the first stage of swallowing.

d **F**— The vagus nerve, through the pharyngeal plexus, is the important innervation. The soft palate is approximated to the pharyngeal wall and closes the pharyngeal isthmus.

e **T**— The larynx is closed off and the pharynx shortened. Respiration is also inhibited during the swallow.

a **F**— The lateral lobes of the gland are related but the isthmus is lower and overlies the 2nd and 3rd tracheal rings.

b **T**

c **T**— The epiglottis and part of the arytenoid cartilage are of this form and do not calcify.

d **T**— From the epiglottis above to the cricoid cartilage below.

e **T**— The geniohyoid and thyrohyoid muscles are innervated by C1 fibres carried in the hypoglossal nerve. In the ansa cervicalis are nerves derived from C2–3 to other infrahyoid muscles.

a **F**— The cricothyroid joints are plane, synovial joints.

b **F**— These ligaments join the thyroid and arytenoid cartilages.

c **T**— The cricothyroid ligament is the anterior edge of this structure.

d **T**— The cricothyroid muscle is innervated by the external

e **T** laryngeal nerve. The other intrinsic muscles are innervated by the recurrent laryngeal nerve.

a **T**— Because of the obliquity of their surfaces downward displacement occurs with lateral gliding.

b **T**— This is the thickened upper border of the conus elasticus. It is covered with mucous membrane and forms the true vocal cord.

c **T**— This thickening in the inferior edge of the aryepiglottic membrane lies within the vestibular fold.

d **F**— This muscle passes from the apex of one arytenoid cartilage to the base of the other as a continuation of the aryepiglottic muscle.

e **T**— Forming an anterior relation of the laryngopharynx.

315 The interior of the larynx:
 a extends into the sinus of the larynx inferior to the
    vocal fold.   (   )
 b is supplied by the recurrent laryngeal nerve up to
    the level of the vestibular fold.   (   )
 c is bounded superiorly by the aryepiglottic folds.   (   )
 d is bounded inferiorly by the rima glottidis.   (   )

 e is lined by stratified squamous epithelium down to
    and including the vocal fold.   (   )

316 In movements of the larynx:
 a forward rotation of the thyroid on the cricoid cartilage
    shortens the vocal folds.   (   )
 b the posterior cricoarytenoid muscles close the vocal
    folds.   (   )
 c the vocalis muscle shortens the fold.   (   )
 d the thyroarytenoid muscle adducts the vocal folds.   (   )
 e contraction of the aryepiglottic muscles approximate
    the vestibular folds.   (   )

317 The external acoustic meatus:
 a is approximately 1.5 cm long.   (   )

 b contains no contribution from the petrous temporal
    bone.   (   )

 c has its medial wall facing downwards and backwards.(   )

 d is innervated posteriorly by the vagus nerve.   (   )

 e is innervated anteriorly by the glossopharyngeal
    nerve.   (   )

318 The middle ear:
 a is lined with stratified squamous epithelium.   (   )

 b communicates with the mastoid antrum through the
    aditus.   (   )
 c is innervated by the mandibular nerve.   (   )

 d accommodates the body of the incus in the
    epitympanic recess.   (   )
 e communicates with the laryngopharynx through the
    auditory tube.   (   )

a F— The sinus lies above the vocal fold between it and the
      vestibular fold and extends up lateral to the vestibular fold.
b F— The internal laryngeal nerve supplies the mucosa over the
      vestibular fold, i.e. including the sinus of the larynx.
c T
d F— This gap between the vocal folds lies above the
      laryngotracheal junction at the cricoid cartilage.
e T— The covering is respiratory epithelium below this level.

a F— The movement, brought about by the cricothyroid muscles,
      lengthens the vocal folds.
b F— These are the only muscles which acting alone can abduct
      the vocal folds.
c T— And also tenses the fold.
d F— This muscle shortens the vocal folds.
e F— This approximates the epiglottis to the arytenoids, closing
      the opening of the larynx.

a F— This approximates only to the cartilaginous lateral third, it
      is about 4 cm long in total.
b T— The bony part of the canal is formed mainly of the
      tympanic part of the temporal bone completed
      posterosuperiorly by the squamous temporal bone.
c F— The lateral surface of the tympanic membrane faces
      downwards and forwards.
d T— The auricular branch of the vagus enters the bone from
      below.
e F— The anterior surface is innervated by the auriculotemporal
      nerve.

a F— Its lining is partly of ciliated columnar and partly of
      squamous epithelium.
b T— Only a thin bony roof separates both cavities from the
      brain.
c F— The innervation is by the glossopharyngeal nerve via the
      tympanic plexus.
d T— The head of the malleus is also situated in this upward
      extension of the cavity.
e F— The communication is with the nasopharynx.

319 **In the middle ear the:**
a facial nerve descends through the anterior wall. ( )

b floor overlies the carotid canal. ( )
c muscle attached to the ossicles are supplied by the vagus nerve. ( )
d foot plate of the stapes overlies the round window (fenestra cochleae). ( )
e the chorda tympani lies on the medial wall. ( )

320 **The cochlea of the bony labyrinth of the internal ear:**
a opens directly into the posterior semicircular canal. ( )

b has a bony medial projection partly dividing its cavity. ( )
c contains the vestibular ganglion within the modiolus. ( )
d contains the scala vestibuli and scala tympani which communicate at the apex of the coil. ( )
e is spirally coiled for $1\frac{1}{2}$ turns. ( )

321 **The membranous labyrinth of the inner ear:**
a is filled with perilymph. ( )

b contains the maculae (organs of balance) within the utricle. ( )
c receives its blood supply from the maxillary artery. ( )

d contains the spiral organ (the organ of hearing) which consists of the hair cells and the tectorial membrane. ( )
e receives proprioceptive fibres from the trigeminal nerve. ( )

322 **The anterior cranial fossa is:**
a limited posteriorly by the squamous temporal bone. ( )
b grooved anteriorly by the inferior sagittal sinus. ( )

c pierced by the nasociliary nerve. ( )

d pierced by the olfactory tracts. ( )

e formed centrally by the body of the sphenoid bone. ( )

a F— The nerve firstly runs backwards along the roof of the cavity and then descends behind the posterior wall.
b T— Also the jugular foramen posteriorly.
c F— The stapedius is supplied by the facial nerve and the tensor tympani by the mandibular nerve.
d F— The foot plate overlies the oval window (fenestra vestibuli).

e F— The nerve lies on the tympanic membrane in the lateral wall.

a F— The anteriorly situated cochlea opens into the vestibule which communicates posteriorly with the semicircular canals.
b T— This is the spiral lamina from the central bony pillar (modiolus).
c F— This ganglion lies in the internal acoustic meatus. The modiolus contains the cochlear ganglion.
d T— The communication is the small opening, the helicotrema.

e F— The coil has $2\frac{3}{4}$ turns around the central bony pillar.

a F— The cavity is filled with endolymph. Perilymph fills the space between the membranous and bony labyrinths.
b T— Maculae are also present within the saccule. The semicircular canals contain the cristae.
c F— Its main supply is from the labyrinthine branch of the basilar artery.
d T— The hair cells support the tectorial membrane and lie on the basilar membrane in the cochlear duct.

e F— The maculae and cristae are innervated by the vestibular division of the 8th cranial nerve.

a F— The lesser wings of the sphenoid from the posterior border.
b F— The vault is grooved by the superior sagittal sinus and the arachnoid granulations on each side.
c F— The anterior ethmoidal vessel and nerve pierce the cribriform plate.
d F— The olfactory tracts and bulbs rest on the floor of the fossa. The olfactory nerves surrounded by their meningeal coverings pierce the cribriform plate and enter the bulb.
e F— The ethmoid plate lies centrally.

323 In the middle cranial fossa the:

a median portion is formed by the body of the sphenoid bone.   (   )

b the internal carotid artery enters through the foramen lacerum.   (   )

c the foramen rotundum transmits the oculomotor nerve.   (   )

d foramen ovale lies within the apex of the petrous temporal bone.   (   )

e foramen spinosum transmits the meningeal branch of the mandibular nerve.   (   )

324 In the posterior cranial fossa the:

a jugular foramen transmits the last three cranial nerves.   (   )

b inferior petrosal sinus grooves the dorsum sellae.   (   )

c sigmoid sinus marks the upper limit of the fossa.   (   )

d jugular foramen lies within the occipital bone.   (   )

e the facial nerve passes across the apex of the petrous temporal bone.   (   )

325 In the cranial nerves:

a special visceral efferent fibres are located in the oculomotor nerve to the eye muscles.   (   )

b special visceral afferent fibres are located in the glossopharyngeal nerve.   (   )

c general visceral afferent fibres are located in the oculomotor nerve.   (   )

d general somatic sensory fibres are located in the glossopharyngeal nerve.   (   )

e general somatic motor fibres are located in the vagus nerve.   (   )

a **T**— The lateral portion is formed by the lesser and greater wings of the sphenoid, and the squamous and petrous parts of the temporal bone.

b **F**— The foramen floors the medial end of the carotid canal which contains the internal carotid artery.

c **F**— The foramen transmits the maxillary nerve, the oculomotor leaves the fossa through the superior orbital fissure.

d **F**— The foramen lies within the greater wing of the sphenoid and transmits the mandibular nerve.

e **T**— Also the middle meningeal vessels.

a **F**— It transmits the glossopharyngeal, vagus and accessory nerves. The hypoglossal passes through the hypoglossal canal in front of the condyle.

b **F**— The sinus descends over the medial end of the petrous temporal bone to the jugular foramen.

c **F**— The transverse sinus marks the upper limit of the fossa. The tentorium cerebelli forms the roof.

d **F**— The foramen lies between the occipital and the petrous temporal bones.

e **F**— The nerve passes into the internal acoustic meatus.

a **F**— The eye muscles, like the tongue, are derived from somatic mesenchyme whereas the special visceral muscle is that derived from the mesenchyme of the pharyngeal arches. It is supplied by the trigeminal, facial, glossopharyngeal and vagus nerves.

b **T**— These are taste fibres. Taste fibres also travel in the facial nerve.

c **T**— These are parasympathetic fibres and are also present in the facial, glossopharyngeal and vagus nerves.

d **F**— The general somatic function is subserved by the trigeminal nerve.

e **F**— These fibres are in the oculomotor, trochlear, abducent and hypoglossal nerves.

326　The olfactory nerves:
a　pierce the cribriform plate of the ethmoid.　( )

b　lie in the wall of the frontal sinus.　( )
c　originate in the bipolar olfactory cells of the olfactory tract.　( )
d　carry a meningeal sheath through the cribriform plate.　( )
e　supply the mucous membrane over the inferior concha.　( )

327　The optic nerve:
a　has its cell bodies in the internal nuclear layer of the retina.　( )
b　has its peripheral endings in the internal plexiform area of the retina.　( )
c　is surrounded by a meningeal sheath containing cerebrospinal fluid up to the eyeball.　( )
d　leaves the orbit through the same foramen as the frontal nerve.　( )
e　passes through the same foramen as the ophthalmic artery.　( )

328　The optic nerve:
a　has the ciliary ganglion on its lateral side.　( )
b　is crossed from lateral to medial by the ophthalmic artery in the orbit.　( )
c　enters the middle cranial fossa lateral to the internal carotid artery.　( )
d　is separated from the pituitary gland by the diaphragma sellae.　( )
e　lies on the sphenoid bone.　( )

329　The oculomotor nerve:
a　supplies the ciliary muscle with general visceral motor fibres.　( )

b　has its nucleus in the periacqueductal grey matter of the midbrain.　( )
c　supplies somatic motor fibres to the superior oblique muscle.　( )
d　divides into superior and inferior divisions near the superior orbital fissure.　( )
e　supplies the inferior oblique muscle.　( )

a **T**— About 15–20 bundles of nerves pierce the cribriform plate on each side and enter the olfactory bulb.

b **F**

c **F**— The bipolar cells lie in the olfactory mucous membrane.

d **T**— Fractures of the cribriform plate allow CSF to escape into the nasal cavity.

e **F**— The olfactory mucosa lines only the upper part of the nasal cavity.

a **F**— This layer contains retinal bipolar cells. The nerve arises in the ganglion layer.

b **T**— Where synapses occur with the bipolar cells.

c **T**— Meninges are carried forward to this level.

d **F**— The optic nerve passes through the optic canal, and the frontal through the supraorbital fissure.

e **T**

a **T**

b **T**— The nasociliary nerve also crosses above the optic nerve.

c **F**— The nerve is medial to the artery and its ophthalmic branch.

d **T**— And the intercavernous sinuses.

e **T**— In its short intracranial portion.

a **T**— These parasympathetic fibres synapse in the ciliary ganglion and supply the sphincter muscle in the ciliary body and the iris.

b **T**— The nucleus lies in the midline in front and in the adjacent grey matter on each side.

c **F**— This muscle is supplied by the trochlear nerve.

d **T**— And supplies all the extraocular muscles except the superior oblique (4th) and lateral rectus (6th).

e **T**— Through its inferior division.

330   The oculomotor nerve:

a   has the longest intracranial course of the ocular
nerves.   (   )

b   pierces the cerebral layer of dura and passes forward
in the lateral wall of the cavernous sinus.   (   )

c   lies at first above and then descends medial to the
trochlear nerve in the cavernous sinus.   (   )

d   when injured, may be associated with dilatation of
the pupil.   (   )

e   passes between the posterior and inferior cerebellar
arteries.   (   )

331   The trochlear nerve:

a   has its nucleus in the lower midbrian.   (   )

b   carries special visceral efferent fibres.   (   )

c   passes between the posterior cerebral and superior
cerebellar arteries.   (   )

d   passes between the oculomotor and ophthalmic
nerves.   (   )

e   passes medially between levator palpebrae
superioris and the roof of the orbit.   (   )

332   The trigeminal nerve:

a   is entirely sensory.   (   )

b   emerges from the brain stem at the upper border
of the pons.   (   )

c   leaves the brain stem as separate sensory and
somatic motor roots.   (   )

d   ganglion is completely surrounded by the meninges. (   )

e   ganglion lies on the body of the sphenoid bone.   (   )

a **F**— The abducent nerve is longer and thinner, and is particularly susceptible to damage in raised intracranial pressure.

b **T**— It is also related to the internal carotid artery, the abducent and trochlear nerves and the ophthalmic nerve in the cavernous sinus.

c **T**

d **T**— This may occur with lateral shift of the brain in head injuries. The patient's eye is deviated and the upper eyelid droops.

e **F**— In the posterior cranial fossa the nerve passes between the posterior cerebral and superior cerebellar arteries.

a **T**— Anterior to the periaqueductal grey matter, the fibres pass posteriorly and undergo a dorsal decussation before emerging.

b **F**— The eye muscles are derived from somatic mesenchyme, so the nerve is classed as a somatic efferent nerve.

c **T**

d **T**— In the lateral wall of the cavernous sinus.

e **T**— And supplies the superior oblique muscle.

a **F**— It is also motor to the muscles of mastication.

b **F**— The nerve leaves the middle of the pons at its junction with the middle cerebellar peduncle.

c **T**— The motor root is separate and carries special visceral motor fibres. It joins the mandibular nerve.

d **F**— The dural sheath (cavum trigeminale) only partly surrounds the ganglion.

e **F**— It lies on the apex of the petrous temporal bone.

333 **The ophthalmic division of the trigeminal nerve transports parasympathetic motor fibres:**

a to the ciliary ganglion. ( )

b from the glossopharyngeal nerve. ( )

c from the facial nerve. ( )

d to the submandibular ganglion. ( )

e to the otic ganglion. ( )

334 **The nasociliary nerve:**

a gives sensory innervation to the medial part of the forehead. ( )

b innervates the eyeball. ( )

c supplies sensory innervation to the dura of the anterior cranial fossa. ( )

d innervates both anterior and posterior ethmoidal air cells. ( )

e innervates the medial part of the upper eyelid. ( )

335 **The maxillary division of the trigeminal nerve:**

a passes through the pterygopalatine fossa. ( )

b innervates all the teeth of the upper jaw. ( )

c innervates the upper anterior quadrant of the lateral wall of the nose. ( )

d innervates the upper posterior quadrant of the lateral wall of the nose. ( )

e innervates the skin of the temple. ( )

a **F**— These come from the oculomotor nerve through its branch to the inferior oblique muscle.

b **F**— The glossopharyngeal fibres run to the otic ganglion and then with the auriculotemporal branch of the mandibular division to the parotid gland.

c **T**— The innervation of the lacrimal gland comes from the facial nerve through the greater petrosal nerve, the pterygopalatine ganglion and the zygomaticotemporal nerve, and then through the lacrimal branch of the ophthalmic nerve.

d **F**— These come from the facial nerve through the chorda tympani and pass with the mandibular division.

e **F**— This receives parasympathetic fibres from the lesser petrosal nerve, the fibres coming from the glossopharyngeal nerve.

a **F**— The supratrochlear and supraorbital branches of the frontal nerve supply this region.

b **T**— Through the long ciliary nerves and the short ciliary nerves (via the ciliary ganglion), carrying sensory fibres from the cornea and sclera. Sympathetic fibres from the internal carotid plexus are also carried.

c **T**— The anterior ethmoidal nerve passes through the medial wall of the orbit on the cribriform plate through which it descends and supplies the nasal cavity and the skin over the nose.

d **T**— Through the anterior and posterior ethmoidal nerves. The posterior also supplies the sphenoidal air sinus.

e **T**— Through the infratrochlear nerve; it also supplies the conjunctiva and a part of the lateral wall of the nose.

a **T**— Entering it through the foramen rotundum. The pterygopalatine ganglion is suspended from the nerve.

b **T**— Through the anterior and posterior superior alveolar nerves.

c **F**— This is supplied by the anterior ethmoidal nerve.

d **T**— By the nasal nerves. The lower half is supplied by the greater palatine and superior alveolar branches of the division.

e **T**— The zygomatic nerve also carries parasympathetic fibres to the lacrimal gland.

336   The mandibular divison of the trigeminal nerve:
  a lies lateral to the otic ganglion.   (   )

  b supplies the levator veli palatine muscle via fibres
      from the medial pterygoid nerve which pass without
      synapsing through the otic ganglion.   (   )
  c innervates the dura of the middle cranial fossa. (   )
  d innervates the posterior part of the tympanic
      membrane.   (   )

  e supplies the buccinator muscle.   (   )

337   The lingual nerve:
  a innervates the lower molar teeth.   (   )
  b innervates the anterior belly of the digastric muscle. (   )

  c passes anterior to the lingula.   (   )

  d carries taste fibres from the circumvalate papillae. (   )

  e carries secretomotor fibres to the parotid gland.   (   )

338   The abducent nerve:
  a has its nucleus in the floor of the 4th ventricle. (   )

  b pierces the inner layer of dura over the dorsum
      sellae.   (   )
  c lies medial to the internal carotid artery in the
      cavernous sinus.   (   )
  d traverses the supraorbital fissure within the
      tendinous ring.   (   )
  e is deeply placed and rarely damaged by intracranial
      disease.   (   )

a **T**— Between tensor veli palatini medially and the lateral pterygoid muscle laterally.

b **F**— Both the tensor tympani and tensor veli palatini muscles are innervated in this fashion. The levator is supplied by the pharyngeal branches of the vagus nerve.

c **T**— A branch passing upwards through the foramen spinosum.

d **F**— The auriculotemporal nerve supplies the anterior part of the membrane and also transports sympathetic and parasympathetic fibres to the parotid gland. The posterior part of the membrane is supplied by the auricular branch of the vagus.

e **F**— This is supplied by the facial nerve. The mandibular nerve supplies the muscles of mastication.

a **F**— All the lower teeth and the anterior belly of the digastric

b **F** and mylohyoid muscles are supplied by the inferior alveolar nerve.

c **T**— It then crosses the root of the 3rd molar tooth before passing between the mylohyoid and hyoglossus muscles.

d **F**— It carries taste and general somatic sensory fibres from the tongue in front of these papillae. Taste fibres together with parasympathetic fibres are carried in the chorda tympani nerve. The glossopharyngeal nerve supplies the circumvallate papillae and the mucous membrane behind them.

e **F**— It carries fibres from the chorda tympani for the submandibular and sublingual salivary glands.

a **T**— The facial fibres arching over it form the facial colliculus in the lower pons above the striae medullaris.

b **T**— Passing anteriorly over the apex of the petrous temporal bone.

c **F**— It is closely related to the lateral surface of the artery within the sinus.

d **T**— And supplies the lateral rectus muscle.

e **F**— Its long intracranial course makes it susceptible to increased intracranial pressure.

339   **The facial nerve:**
- **a**   ganglion (geniculate) contains the cell bodies of its parasympathetic fibres.   (   )
- **b**   carries secretomotor fibres from the lower part of the salivary nucleus.   (   )
- **c**   has its taste and secretomotor fibres as a separate nerve in the internal acoustic meatus.   (   )
- **d**   leaves the skull through the mastoid foramen.   (   )
- **e**   lies medial to the external carotid artery.   (   )

340   **The facial nerve:**
- **a**   has a branch containing parasympathetic fibres leaving it at the facial ganglion.   (   )
- **b**   has a branch, passing through the petrotympanic fissure, and then supplying the 1st pharyngeal arch muscle.   (   )
- **c**   passes medial to the styloid process.   (   )
- **d**   carries secretomotor fibres to the parotid gland.   (   )
- **e**   innervates the temporalis muscle.   (   )

341   **The vestibulocochlear nerve:**
- **a**   is formed at the base of the modiolus.   (   )
- **b**   lies posterior to the facial nerve in the internal acoustic meatus.   (   )
- **c**   enters the cerebellomedullary angle of the brain stem.   (   )
- **d**   has its central nuclei in the anterior pons.   (   )
- **e**   passes into the middle cranial fossa over the apex of the posterior temporal bone.   (   )

a **F**— This is a sensory ganglion mainly for taste fibres passing to the nucleus of the tractus solitarius.

b **F**— These parasympathetic fibres arise in the upper part of the salivary nucleus in the medulla.

c **T**— The nervus intermedius joins the main trunk near the facial ganglion.

d **F**— This foramen transmits an emissary vein. The nerve passes through the stylomastoid foramen.

e **F**— It lies lateral to the artery within the parotid gland.

a **T**— The greater petrosal nerve passes through the petrous temporal bone and becomes the nerve of the pterygoid canal, before reaching the pterygopalatine ganglion where its fibres synapse.

b **F**— The facial nerve supplies 2nd pharyngeal arch muscle but its chorda tympani branch, passing through the petrotympanic fissure, carries taste and parasympathetic fibres to 1st arch derivates.

c **F**— The nerve passes lateral to the styloid process on its way into the parotid gland.

d **F**— The parotid gland receives parasympathetic fibres from the glossopharyngeal nerve via the lesser petrosal nerve, the otic ganglion and the auriculotemporal nerve. The secretomotor fibres in the facial nerve pass mainly to the submandibular and sublingual glands via the submandibular ganglion.

e **F**— Its motor fibres are predominantly to the muscles of facial expression.

a **F**— The vestibular and cochlear parts unite in the internal acoustic meatus where the vestibular ganglion is situated. The cochlear ganglion is in the modiolus.

b **T**

c **T**— Lying lateral to the facial nerve.

d **F**— The vestibular nuclei lie in the floor of the 4th ventricle, and the cochlear nuclei in the floor of the lateral recess of the 4th ventricle.

e **F**— The nerve endings are situated within the petrous temporal bone and the nerve passes into the posterior cranial fossa.

342 The glossopharyngeal nerve carries:
  a fibres from the nucleus ambiguus.   (   )
  b somatic motor fibres.   (   )

  c fibres to the nucleus of the tractus solitarius.   (   )

  d fibres from the lower part of the salivary nucleus.   (   )

  e general visceral sensory fibres.   (   )

343 The vagus nerve carries:
  a fibres from the nucleus ambiguus.   (   )
  b somatic motor fibres.   (   )
  c fibres to the nucleus of the tractus solitarius.   (   )

  d fibres from the upper salivary nucleus.   (   )

  e somatic sensory fibres.   (   )

344 The vagus nerve:
  a crosses the left subclavian artery in the root of
     the neck.   (   )

  b carries general visceral sensory fibres.   (   )

  c leaves the skull between the internal jugular vein
     posteriorly and the inferior petrosal sinus anteriorly.   (   )
  d leaves the medulla as a number of rootlets between
     the olive and pyramid.   (   )
  e lies posterolateral to the common carotid artery.   (   )

a T— Special visceral motor fibres supply the stylopharyngeus
b F   muscle. These are the only fibres to voluntary muscle in
         the nerve.
c T— Special visceral sensory fibres carry taste from the
         posterior third of the tongue.
d T— General visceral motor fibres relay in the otic ganglion and
         pass to the parotid gland.
e T— From the middle ear, pharynx, palate, posterior third of
         tongue, carotid sinus and carotid body.

a T— Special visceral motor fibres supply the striated muscle of
b F   the larynx, pharynx and palate.
c T— Special visceral sensory fibres carry tastes from the
         valleculae and the epiglottis.
d F— The parasympathetic (general visceral motor) fibres supply
         the heart, the lungs and the alimentary tract as far as the
         splenic flexure.
e T— From the posterior part of the external acoustic meatus
         and the tympanic membrane by its auricular branch.

a F— This is the relation of the right side, but on the left the
         nerve descends between the subclavian and common
         carotid arteries.
b T— From the mucous membrane of the palate, pharynx, larynx
         and also from the heart, lungs and alimentary tract.
c T— And between the glossopharyngeal nerve anteriorly, and
         the accessory nerve posteriorly in the jugular foramen.
d F— The rootlets lie lateral to the olive. In the jugular foramen
         and just below it are the two sensory ganglia of the vagus.
e T— With the internal jugular vein, within the carotid sheath.

345   The spinal accessory nerve:
a   carries somatic motor fibres to the sterno-
      cleidomastoid muscle.   (   )
b   carries the special visceral motor fibres to the
      trapezius muscle.   (   )

c   spinal root ascends behind the ligamenta denticulata. (   )
d   passes laterally behind the jugular vein over the
      transverse process of the atlas.   (   )
e   lies medial to the vagus nerve.   (   )

346   The hypoglossal nerve:
a   emerges, from the medulla, between the pyramid
      and the olive.   (.)
b   passes anteriorly deep to the posterior belly of the
      digastric muscle.   (   )
c   passes forwards between the internal and external
      carotid arteries.   (   )
d   carries fibres of the 1st cervical nerve to the
      geniohyoid muscle.   (   )
e   is crossed by the submandibular duct.   (   )

347   The cervical fascia splits:
a   and embraces the infrahyoid muscles.   (   )

b   and partially encloses the submandibular salivary
      gland.   (   )
c   inferiorly enclosing the jugular venous arch.   (   )
d   posteriorly around the scapula.   (   )

e   to enclose the sternocleidomastoid muscle.   (   )

348   The prevertebral fascia:
a   encloses the thyroid gland.   (   )

b   extends laterally into the upper limb as the axillary
      sheath.   (   )
c   has the cervical sympathetic chain embedded in it. (   )
d   blends inferiorly with the anterior longitudinal
      ligament in front of the body of the 6th cervical
      vertebra.   (   )
e   splits around the hyoid bone.   (   )

a T— These fibres arise in the upper five cervical segments of the cord.

b F— The cranial root of the nerve carries special visceral fibres which join the vagus. The somatic motor fibres supply the sternocleidomastoid and trapezius muscles.

c T— As it represents a dorsal root nerve.

d F— The nerve passes in front of the vein.

e F— It lies lateral to the vagus as they leave the skull through the jugular foramen.

a T— The nucleus lies in the floor of the 4th ventricle on each side of the midline.

b T— Lying at first on the middle constrictor and then on the hyoglossus muscle.

c F— The nerve passes lateral and then anterior to both vessels and to the loop of the lingual artery.

d T— Also to the thyrohyoid, and to the strap muscles via the superior root of the ansa cervicalis.

e F— The duct has a close relationship to the lingual nerve.

a F— These infrahyoid muscles are embedded in its deep surface.

b T— It also splits and forms the covering of the parotid gland.

c T— In the region of the manubrial attachment of the fascia.

d F— It is attached to the ligamentum nuchae above and to the spine of the scapula. Below the scapula it is continuous with the thoracolumbar fascia.

e T— Also the trapezius.

a F— The pretracheal fascia encloses the gland blending inferiorly with the adventitia of the great vessels.

b T— The subclavian artery and the brachial plexus carry the fascia into the axilla.

c T— The chain lies posterior to the carotid sheath.

d F— It extends to the level of the 4th thoracic vertebra.

e F— The hyoid receives the superior attachment of the pretracheal fascia.

349   The carotid sheath:
  a   is attached superiorly to the base of skull.   (   )
  b   fuses with the pericardium inferiorly.   (   )
  c   lies deep to the prevertebral fascia.   (   )
  d   encloses the jugular vein and vagus nerve.   (   )
  e   encloses the external carotid artery.   (   )

350   The posterior triangle of the neck:
  a   is floored by the prevertebral fascia.   (   )

  b   is bordered posteriorly by the rhomboideus major
      muscle.   (   )
  c   has the spine of the scapula as its inferior border.   (   )
  d   is bordered anteriorly by the sternocleidomastoid
      muscle.   (   )
  e   is crossed by the internal jugular vein.   (   )

351   The sternocleidomastoid muscle:
  a   is innervated by the 2nd and 3rd cervical nerve
      roots.   (   )
  b   is surrounded by the cervical fascia.   (   )

  c   is attached superiorly along the lateral half of the
      superior nuchal line.   (   )
  d   acting with its fellow of the opposite side, retracts
      the face.   (   )

  e   has a single inferior attachment to the upper medial
      third of the clavicle.   (   )

352   The semispinalis capitis muscle is:
  a   attached superiorly to the mastoid process and the
      lateral part of the superior nuchal line.   (   )

  b   superfical to levatores costarum.   (   )

  c   mainly concerned with the maintenance of the
      upright position.   (   )
  d   supplied by the dorsal rami of the spinal nerves.   (   )
  e   a medial relation of the suboccipital triangle.   (   )

a T— It is a condensation of the fascias of the neck and below
b T   fuses with the fibrous pericardium.
c F— It lies anterior to the prevertebral fascia.
d T
e F— It encloses the common and internal carotid arteries.

a T— Overlying the splenius capitis, levator scapulae and scalenus medius muscles.
b F— The posterior border is formed by the trapezius muscle.
c F— The middle third of the clavicle forms the inferior border.
d T— The posterior border of this muscle forms the anterior limit of the triangle.
e F— It is crossed by the external jugular vein, accessory nerve and omohyoid muscle.

a T— Directly, but mainly through fibres carried in the spinal accessory nerve.
b T— The fascia splits anteriorly and encloses this muscle and posteriorly for trapezius.
c T— And to the mastoid process.
d F— Together they protrude the face. One muscle turns the face towards the opposite side and also rotates the face, raising the chin.
e F— A second head is attached to the anterior surface of the manubrium sterni.

a F— These are the attachments of the splenius capitis deep to sternocleidomastoid. Semispinalis is attached between the superior and inferior nuchal lines nearer the midline.
b T— The latter, like the multifidus, rotatores, interspinous and intertransversus muscles, are part of the deep short muscle system.
c T— It is an antigravity muscle.
d T— As are most muscles in this region of the trunk and neck.
e F— It lies superficial to the suboccipital triangle.

353   The suboccipital triangle:

a   is bounded laterally by the rectus capitis posterior major muscle.   (   )

b   is bounded inferiorly by the inferior oblique muscle. (   )
c   is crossed superficially by the greater occipital nerve. (   )

d   has the posterior atlanto-occipital membrane in its floor.   (   )
e   is bounded by muscles which extend and rotate the head on the cervical vertebrae.   (   )

354   The scalenus anterior muscle:

a   is attached superiorly to the bodies of the 3rd–6th cervical vertebrae.   (   )
b   is attached inferiorly to the anterior border of the 1st rib.   (   )
c   lies anterior to the subclavian vein on the 1st rib.   (   )

d   is crossed anteriorly by the phrenic nerve.   (   )

e   forms the posterior relation of the roots of the brachial plexus.   (   )

355   The omohyoid muscle:

a   is attached superiorly to the greater horn of the hyoid bone.   (   )
b   is attached by its intermediate tendon to the scapula. (   )

c   crosses over the external jugular vein.   (   )
d   crosses over the scalenus anterior muscle.   (   )

e   crosses the accessory nerve.   (   )

a F— This muscle passes from the spine of the axis to the occipital bone below the inferior nuchal line and forms the medial border of the triangle.

b T— The superior oblique forms the lateral boundary.

c T— And covered by the semispinalis and longissimus capitis muscles.

d T— The vertebral artery and 1st cervical nerve pass beneath it.

e T— They probably are involved in the small movements necessary in centring the visual axes, important in stereoscopic vision.

a F— It is attached to the anterior tubercles on the transverse processes of these vertebrae.

b F— The scalene tubercle is on the medial border of the rib.

c F— The vein lies anterior; the subclavian artery and the T1 root of the brachial plexus lie posterior.

d T— The nerve descends along its medial border, deep to the prevertebral fascia, crosses over the muscle, and then enters the thorax.

e F— These nerves lie deep to the muscle.

a F— It is attached to the body of the bone.

b F— The inferior belly is attached to the superior border of the scapula. The tendon is attached to the medial end of the clavicle by a fascial sling.

c F— It lies anterior to the internal jugular vein.

d T— Separated by the contents of the carotid sheath and the phrenic nerve.

e F— The muscle and nerve run parallel courses as they cross the posterior triangle of the neck.

356   The thyroid gland:

a   is limited superiorly by the attachment of the
      sternohyoid muscle.   (   )

b   has the recurrent laryngeal nerve ascending medial
      to the lateral lobes.   (   )

c   develops from a midline ventral diverticulum between
      the 2nd and 3rd pharyngeal arches.   (   )

d   is enclosed in the pretracheal fascia.   (   )

e   receives a major blood supply from the middle
      thyroid artery.   (   )

357   The parathyroid glands:

a   lie between the thyroid gland and the trachea.   (   )

b   receive a rich blood supply from the superior and
      inferior thyroid arteries.   (   )

c   develop eosinophil staining cells around puberty.   (   )

d   develop from a 3rd and 4th pharyngeal arch
      mesenchyme.   (   )

e   are usually 6–8 mm across.

358   The trachea:

a   divides at the level of the lower border of the 4th
      thoracic vertebra (the sternal angle).   (   )

b   is reinforced by 15–20 complete cartilaginous rings.   (   )

c   is a posterior relation of the jugular venous arch.   (   )

d   is a medial relation of the carotid sheath and its
      contents.   (   )

e   is a posterior relation of the isthmus of the thyroid
      gland.   (   )

a **F**— The upper limit is the oblique line on the thyroid cartilage to which the sternothyroid muscle is attached.

b **T**— The nerve is an important relation in surgical procedures on the gland as it accompanies the inferior thyroid vessels.

c **F**— The diverticulum starts between the 1st and 2nd arches and its position is marked by the foramen caecum on the tongue. The 4th pharyngeal pouch also contributes specialised C-cells to the gland.

d **T**— The gland has also a surface capsule within which is the venous plexus.

e **F**— This artery does not exist; the superior and inferior thyroid arteries require identification and ligation during thyroidectomy.

a **F**— They are situated on the posterior surface of the thyroid gland within its capsule.

b **T**— The presence of these vessels may help to differentiate the glands from fat lobules in surgical procedures.

c **T**— In addition to the columns of chief cells which are separated by blood spaces. The chief cells have dark staining nuclei and a chromatin network.

d **F**— The superior and inferior glands develop respectively from the 4th and 3rd pharyngeal pouch endoderm.

e **F**— They are 3–6 mm and are easily mistaken for fat globules.

a **T**— It begins below the cricoid cartilage, i.e. C6 level.

b **F**— The plates of cartilage are incomplete posteriorly where the trachea rests on the oesophagus. The gap is closed by fibroelastic tissue and smooth muscle.

c **T**— This is an important relation when a tracheotomy is being performed.

d **T**— Behind the carotid sheath is the sympathetic trunk medially with the vertebral and inferior thyroid arteries.

e **T**— This can be palpated over the 2nd and 3rd tracheal rings; it is an important relation in tracheotomy.

359   The oesophagus:
  a   commences about 25 cm from the incisor teeth.   (   )

  b   receives a parasympathetic innervation from the
        greater splanchnic nerve.   (   )

  c   has smooth muscle forming its longitudinal and
        circular muscle coats.   (   )
  d   has numerous mucous glands extending into the
        vascular submucosa.   (   )
  e   has a venous drainage to both portal and systemic
        circulations.   (   )

360   The right subclavian artery:
  a   is formed behind the right sternoclavicular joint.   (   )
  b   passes laterally over the suprapleural membrane.   (   )

  c   terminates at the medial border of the 1st rib.   (   )

  d   lies posterior to the right internal jugular vein.   (   )

  e   is separated from its vein by the scalenus anterior
        muscle.   (   )

361   The left subclavian artery:
  a   is crossed posteriorly by the recurrent laryngeal
        nerve.   (   )
  b   passes anterior to the thoracic duct.   (   )

  c   gives rise to the costocervical trunk medial to the
        scalenus anterior muscle.   (   )
  d   crosses the left sympathetic chain.   (   )

  e   has the vagus on its lateral side.   (   )

a F— The distance in the adult is about 15 cm, the organ being approximately 25 cm long.

b F— This nerve provides a sympathetic innervation. The vagus provides parasympathetic innervation through the recurrent laryngeal nerves to the upper part and through the oesophageal plexus to the lower part. Within the recurrent laryngeal nerve are special visceral motor fibres to the striated muscle.

c T— Although the upper third is composed mainly of striated muscle, there is a little smooth muscle.

d T— The glands are less prominent in the upper than the lower end of the oesophagus and are almost absent in the middle.

e T— These communications may enlarge in liver disease.

a T— The left artery arises directly from the arch of the aorta.

b T— The membrane separates the artery from the pleura and the apex of the lung.

c F— The subclavian artery becomes the axillary artery at the outer border of the first rib.

d T— The vein and the vagus nerve descend in front of the artery in the root of the neck.

e T— The subclavian vein lies anterior to the prevertebral fascia and its tributaries lie outside the axillary sheath.

a F— On the right side the nerve hooks back around the artery but on the left it passes back around the arch of the aorta.

b F— The duct passes in front of the artery and enters the origin of the left brachiocephalic vein.

c T— On the right side this usually occurs behind the muscle.

d F— The dome of the pleura and the apex of the lung separate the vessel from the neck of the 1st rib where the sympathetic chain is found.

e F— The vagus and phrenic nerves lie medially, between the subclavian and common carotid arteries.

362   The vertebral artery:
a   arises from the subclavian artery medial to scalenus anterior.   (   )
b   is a posterior relation of the common carotid artery. (   )
c   is surrounded by a sympathetic plexus derived from the inferior cervical sympathetic ganglion.   (   )
d   enters the foramen tranversarium of the 6th cervical vertebra.   (   )
e   has the dorsal ramus of the 1st cervical nerve between it and the transverse mass of the atlas.   (   )

363   The thyrocervical trunk:
a   gives rise to the deep cervical artery.   (   )
b   gives rise to the internal thoracic artery.   (   )
c   sends a blood supply to the thyroid gland.   (   )
d   divides at the level of the thyroid isthmus.   (   )
e   is crossed by the phrenic nerve on the right side.   (   )

364   The common carotid artery:
a   terminates at the level of the upper border of the thyroid cartilage.   (   )
b   is a posterolateral relation to the thyroid gland.   (   )
c   is crossed anterolaterally by the omohyoid muscle.   (   )
d   is crossed anterolaterally by the sternocleidomastoid muscle.   (   )
e   at its bifurcation, has baro- and chemoreceptors which are richly innervated by the glossopharyngeal nerve. (   )

a **T**— As do the thyrocervical trunk and internal thoracic artery.

b **T**— It is also crossed by the inferior thyroid artery.
c **T**— The sympathetic nerves are distributed with the branches of the vertebral and basilar arteries.
d **T**— The artery has a very tortuous course. After passing through the foramen magnum it joins its fellow of the
e **T** opposite side and forms the basilar artery. It supplies most of the hindbrain and the medial aspect of the occipital pole of the cerebral hemisphere (visual area).

a **F**— The deep cervical and the highest intercostal arteries are branches of the costocervical trunk.
b **F**— This is a separate branch of the subclavian artery.
c **T**— Through its inferior thyroid branch.
d **F**— The short trunk soon divides into inferior thyroid, transverse cervical and suprascapular arteries.
e **F**— The transverse cervical and suprascapular branches of the trunk cross anterior to the nerve.

a **T**

b **T**— The thyroid gland may be an ant∍rior or a medial relation to the artery.
c **T**— It is accompanied by the vagus nerve and the internal
d **T**— jugular vein. All are surrounded by the carotid sheath and crossed anterolaterally by the sternocleidomastoid muscle.
e **T**— They are also innervated from the cervical sympathetic trunk.

365   The exterenal carotid artery:
a   terminates by dividing into superficial temporal and
transverse facial arteries.   (   )
b   lies lateral to the retromandibular vein.   (   )

c   has all the styloid muscles passing between it and
the internal carotid artery.   (   )
d   is crossed medially by the lingual nerve.   (   )
e   lies deep to the hypoglossal nerve.   (   )

366   The facial artery:
a   is crossed laterally by the hypoglossal nerve.   (   )

b   is a branch of the maxillary artery.   (   )
c   grooves the inferior surface of the submandibular
gland.   (   )
d   passes medially over the middle and superior
constrictor muscles.   (   )
e   traverses the face between the superficial and deep
muscles.   (   )

367   The maxillary artery:
a   lies betweeen the neck of the mandible and the
sphenomandibular ligament.   (   )
b   passes through the infratemporal fossa.   (   )

c   traverses the sphenopalatine canal.   (   )
d   sends branches to the lateral wall of the nose.   (   )

e   sends a branch through the foramen spinosum.   (   )

368   The middle meningeal artery:
a   passes through the foramen ovale.   (   )
b   lies in the anterior cranial fossa.   (   )
c   lies in intimate relationship with the skull.   (   )
d   lies deep to the zygomaticofrontal suture.   (   )

e   also supplies the diploë.   (   )

a **F**— The superficial temporal and maxillary arteries are the terminal divisions, being formed behind the neck of the mandible.

b **F**— The artery lies medial to the vein and the facial nerve in the parotid gland.

c **F**— The stylohyoid passes lateral to both vessels. The process, styloglossus and stylopharyngeus pass between the vessels.

d **F**— The nerve runs in a more anterior plane than the artery.

e **T** Both internal and external carotids are crossed superficially by the facial nerve above and the hypoglossal nerve below.

a **F**— The nerve crosses the loop of the lingual artery inferior to the facial artery.

b **F**— It is a branch of the external carotid artery.

c **F**— The superior surface of the gland is grooved by the artery.

d **T**— Before reaching the deep surface of the submandibular gland.

e **T**— Supplying the upper and lower lips and facial musculature. It crosses the body of the mandible just in front of masseter muscle.

a **T**— The middle meningeal and inferior alveolar arteries arise from the first part of the main vessel.

b **T**— On the lateral surface of the lateral pterygoid muscle. It supplies all the muscles of mastication.

c **F**— It ends in the pterygopalatine fossa and some of its

d **T** terminal branches accompany the branches of the pterygopalatine ganglion.

e **T**— The middle meningeal artery enters the skull and divides. Its anterior branch lies medial to the pterion and is of surgical importance in skull fractures.

a **F**— It gains the middle cranial fossa by ascending through the

b **F** foramen spinosum and lies close to the skull, often

c **T** grooving its inner surface.

d **F**— Its surface marking, of importance for surgical access, is 3.5 cm behind and 1.5 cm above the zygomaticofrontal suture.

e **T**— The vessels are easily damaged in injuries to the skull and may cause a life-threatening haemorrhage.

369   The internal carotid artery:
  a   enters the skull and then divides into the middle
       and posterior cerebral arteries.   (   )

  b   is separated from the external carotid artery by the
       glossopharyngeal nerve.   (   )
  c   is crossed laterally by the posterior belly of the
       digastric muscle.   (   )
  d   is crossed laterally by the facial nerve.   (   )
  e   within the cavernous sinus is related to the
       mandibular nerve.   (   )

370   The internal carotid artery:
  a   lies in the floor of the inner ear.   (   )

  b   grooves the lesser wing of the sphenoid bone.   (   )

  c   lies lateral to the abducent nerve.   (   )
  d   pierces the diaphragma sellae medial to the anterior
       clinoid process.   (   )
  e   sends a branch through the optic canal.   (   )

371   The internal jugular vein:
  a   is a continuation of the transverse cranial venous
       sinus.   (   )
  b   receives the inferior petrosal sinus just below the
       base of the skull.   (   )
  c   has the last four cranial nerves as medial relations
       at the base of the skull.   (   )
  d   is crossed laterally by the hypoglossal nerve.   (   )

  e   lies anterolateral to the sympathetic chain.   (   )

372   The internal jugular vein:
  a   is crossed posteriorly by the accessory nerve.   (   )

  b   lies medial to the styloid process and its muscles.   (   )

  c   is crossed anteriorly from lateral to medial by the
       phrenic nerve in the root of the neck.   (   )
  d   receives the anterior jugular vein.   (   )

  e   lies posterior to the subclavian artery.   (   )

a **F**— It divides into the anterior and middle cerebral arteries. It gives off no branches in the neck. The middle cerebral artery supplies the sensorimotor areas of the cerebral cortex.
b **T**— Also the styloglossus and the stylopharyngeus muscles and the pharyngeal branches of the vagus.
c **T**— Also the stylohyoid muscle.

d **T**— Also the hypoglossal nerve.
e **F**— It is related to the ophthalmic (and maxillary) nerves and the oculomotor, trochlear and abducent nerves.

a **F**— The carotid canal is in the floor of the middle ear and the artery passes anteromedially over the foramen lacerum.
b **F**— The carotid groove is on the body of the sphenoid as the artery lies in the cavernous sinus.
c **F**— The nerve is on its lateral side.
d **T**— The optic nerve and chiasma lie medial to the artery.

e **T**— The ophthalmic artery lies lateral to the nerve in the canal and later gives off the central artery of the retina.

a **F**— It is a continuation of the sigmoid sinus through the base of the skull.
b **T**— The 9th, 10th and 11th cranial nerves lie between the two vessels in the jugular foramen.
c **T**— The hypoglossal nerve is posteromedial to the other three.

d **F**— The nerve passes forwards medial to the vein and lateral to the internal and external carotid arteries.
e **T**— Separated by the prevertebral fascia.

a **T**— The nerve then passes over the transverse process of the atlas and enters the deep surface of the sternocleidomastoid muscle.
b **T**— Below this level it lies deep to the sternocleidomastoid muscle and is crossed by the posterior belly of the digastric and then by the omohyoid muscles.
c **F**— The nerve lies posterior to the vein.

d **F**— This vein usually passes to the external jugular which enters into the subclavian vein.
e **F**— The artery passes posterior to the vein.

373   The cervical plexus:

a   gives off the greater occipital nerve from the second
     root of the plexus.   (   )

b   gives branches to the skin over the outer part of the
     shoulder.   (   )

c   supplies the inferior part of the external acoustic
     meatus.   (   )
d   lies deep to scalenus anterior muscle.   (   )

e   supplies the thyrohyoid muscle.   (   )

374   The phrenic nerve:

a   is mainly derived from the 4th cervical nerve root.   (   )
b   lies deep to the prevertebral fascia.   (   )

c   passes anterior to the subclavian artery on the left
     side.   (   )
d   crosses anterior to the internal thoracic artery, at the
     inlet of the thorax.   (   )
e   passes anterior to the subclavian vein.   (   )

375   The superior cervical ganglion:

a   lies between the prevertebral fascia and the internal
     jugular vein.   (   )

b   gives rise to the cardiac branches.   (   )

c   gives rise to the deep petrosal nerve.   (   )
d   when damaged gives rise to a Horner's syndrome.   (   )

e   gives rise to the ansa subclavia.   (   )

a **F**— This large nerve is derived from the dorsal ramus of the second cervical nerve. The cervical plexus is formed from ventral rami of cervical nerves.

b **T**— The phrenic nerve (C3, 4 & 5) supplies the diaphragm which has 'migrated down' during embryonic development. The supraclavicular nerves come from the same segments, and pain may be referred from the diaphragm to the shoulder region.

c **F**— The great auricular nerves (C2 and 3) supply the skin over the inferior auricle but not the meatus.

d **T**— On scalenus medius. The roots of the brachial plexus also lie between these two scalene muscles.

e **T**— This and the geniohyoid muscle are supplied by C1 fibres carried by the hypoglossal nerve.

a **T**— It is usually supplemented by C3 and C5 fibres.

b **T**— Passing on to the anterior surface of the scalenus anterior muscle.

c **T**— It is placed more laterally on the right side and separated from the artery by the scalenus anterior muscle.

d **T**

e **F**— The nerve lies posterior to the subclavian vein.

a **T**— It lies in the fascia on the 2nd and 3rd cervical transverse processes, deep to the angle of the mandible, and posteromedial to the vein.

b **T**— Cardiac branches arise from all three cervical sympathetic ganglia.

c **T**— From the plexus it forms around the internal carotid artery.

d **T**— With a drooping upper eyelid, small pupil and loss of sweating from that side of the face.

e **F**— The ansa subclavia passes between the middle and inferior ganglia.

376   The pterygopalatine ganglion:
  a supplies the sphincter pupillae muscle through its
     zygomaticotemporal fibres.   ( )

  b supplies secretomotor fibres to the lacrimal gland. ( )
  c gives passage to sympathetic fibres.   ( )

  d distributes secretomotor fibres to the glands of the
     nose, palate and nasopharynx.   ( )
  e receives fibres from the maxillary nerve.   ( )

377   The submandibular ganglion:
  a distributes secretomotor fibres to the sublingual
     gland.   ( )
  b distributes fibres from the lesser petrosal nerve to
     the submandibular gland.   ( )

  c gives passage to taste fibres from the circumvallate
     papillae.   ( )
  d is situated medial to the hyoglossus muscle.   ( )

  e is closely related to the mandibular nerve.   ( )

378   The lymph drainage of the head and neck:
  a includes a chain of lymph nodes around the
     nasopharynx.   ( )
  b includes a circular chain of lymph nodes around the
     base of the skull.   ( )
  c has a deep cervical lymph chain situated around the
     external and the anterior jugular veins.   ( )

  d on the left side passes via the carotid lymph duct
     into the thoracic duct.   ( )
  e on the right side passes into the right jugular or
     subclavian vein.   ( )

a **F**— This muscle receives fibres from an oculomotor branch to the inferior oblique muscle. The postganglionic fibres arise in the ciliary ganglion.

b **T**— Via the zygomaticotemporal and lacrimal nerves.

c **T**— From the superior cervical ganglion along the plexus around the internal carotid artery, the deep petrosal nerve and the nerve of the pterygoid canal.

d **T**— The preganglionic fibres come in the greater petrosal nerve and the nerve of the pterygoid canal from the facial nerve.

e **T**— The ganglion is suspended from the maxillary nerve, sensory fibres from the nerve are distributed through branches of the ganglion to the nose, palate and nasopharynx.

a **T**— Also to the submandibular gland. The fibres come via the chorda tympani and lingual nerves.

b **F**— The lesser petrosal nerve is derived from the glossopharyngeal tympanic plexus and is distributed to the parotid gland via the otic ganglion and auriculotemporal nerve.

c **F**— These pass to the glossopharyngeal nerve.

d **F**— It is suspended from the lingual nerve on the lateral surface of the muscle.

e **F**

a **T**— Large aggregations of lymph tissue surround this region as the tubal, pharyngeal, palatine and lingual tonsils.

b **T**— The nodes are arranged from the submental group in front to the occipital group behind.

c **F**— The superficial cervical lymph chains lie around these vessels. The deep chain is situated around the internal jugular vein.

d **F**— On the left side, the thoracic duct receives the left jugular lymph trunk. The right jugular duct opens directly into the

e **T** jugular or subclavian vein or into the right lymph duct.

IX Central Nervous System

379   In the central nervous system the:
a   telencephalon comprises the two cerebral
    hemispheres.   (   )

b   rhombencephalon does not include the cerebellum.   (   )
c   brain stem extends from the forebrain to the spinal
    cord.   (   )

d   thalamus is part of the mesencephalon.   (   )
e   hypothalamus is part of the diencephalon.   (   )

380   In the attachment of the cranial nerves the:
a   olfactory bulbs represent a part of the primitive
    forebrain.   (   )
b   oculomotor nerves emerge from the
    interpeduncular fossa.   (   )
c   trochlear nerve emerges dorsally between the
    superior and inferior colliculi.   (   )
d   abducent nerve emerges lateral to the facial and
    vestibulocochlear nerves.   (   )
e   vagus emerges between the olive and the pyramids.   (   )

381   The neural crest tissue:
a   is derived from the neural plate.   (   )

b   contributes to the developing alar lamina.   (   )
c   gives rise to the autonomic ganglia.   (   )
d   gives rise to the cortex of the suprarenal gland.   (   )

e   gives rise to the marginal layer of the neural tube. (   )

a **T**— With the diencephalon (mainly thalamus and hypothalamus) it completes the forebrain (prosencephalon).

b **F**— It consists of the pons, medulla and cerebellum.

c **T**— It consists of the midbrain, pons and medulla. It gives attachment to the cerebellum posteriorly but the cerebellum is excluded.

d **F**— The thalamus and hypothalamus make up most of the

e **T** diencephalon. The mesencephalon is the midbrain.

a **T**— The olfactory bulb and tract, and the optic nerve, are forebrain derivatives.

b **T**— Just posterior to the mamillary bodies.

c **F**— The nuclei lie ventrally in the lower midbrain, but the nerves emerge dorsally below the inferior colliculi.

d **F**— The abducent nerve arises near the midline and medial to the other two nerves.

e **F**— This is site of exit of the hypoglossal nerve; the vagus and cranial nerves emerge between the olive and the inferior cerebellar peduncle.

a **F**— The neural crest tissue is derived from the junctional zone between neural plate ectoderm and embryonic ectoderm.

b **F**— This is a derivative of neural plate ectoderm.

c **T**— Also to the spinal and cranial nerve ganglia.

d **F**— The medulla of the gland is derived from neural crest tissue.

e **F**— The neural tube and its marginal layer are derivatives of neural plate ectoderm.

382 In the development of the spinal cord the:
a ependymal layer lines the cavity in the spinal cord.   (   )
b outer mantle layer contains mainly the nerve fibres.   (   )

c basal (ventral) lamina disappears.   (   )

d autonomic neurons develop adjacent to the sulcus
   limitans.   (   )

e alar (dorsal) lamina give rise to neurons subserving
   motor function.   (   )

383 In the development of the brain:
a a ventral flexure is present at the junction with the
   spinal cord.   (   )
b the ventral flexure precedes the development of
   the dorsal pontine flexure.   (   )
c the cerebellum develops from the rostral edge of
   the roof of the hindbrain vesicle.   (   )
d a single constriction in the neural tube separates it
   into the two primitive vesicles.   (   )
e in the region of the midbrain the alar laminae come
   to lie lateral to the basal laminae.   (   )

384 In the development of the forebrain:
a the basal lamina expands on the ventral aspect of
   the forebrain vesicle.   (   )
b the hippocampus develops on the medial surface
   of the hemisphere dorsal to the interventricular
   foramen.   (   )
c the piriform cortex develops on the medial surface
   of the hemisphere, ventral to the interventricular
   foramen.   (   )
d commissural fibres from the piriform cortex pass
   through the lamina terminalis.   (   )
e the fornix commissure connects the two thalami.   (   )

a T— Although this cavity is poorly developed in the adult.

b F— The mantle layer is the intermediate layer containing the bodies of the neuroblasts. The outer (marginal) layer contains mainly fibres.

c F— The basal lamina gives rise to the neurons subserving motor function.

d T— The sulcus separates the ventral motor and the dorsal sensory areas. The visceral neurons adjacent to the sulcus form the lateral horn of grey matter which is prominent in the thoracic and sacral regions.

e F— They give rise to sensory neurons.

a T— This is the spinal flexure.

b T— As does the spinal flexure.

c T— At first growing into the vesicle but later becoming everted and undergoing external enlargement.

d F— Two constrictions occur and divide it into the three primitive vesicles of the forebrain, midbrain and hindbrain.

e F— This arrangement does occur in the region of the pontine flexure. Additional columns of neurons — special visceral (branchial) — are present in the brain stem, carrying taste fibres and supplying pharyngeal arch musculature.

a F— The basal lamina is absent. The forebrain develops from the alar lamina.

b T— With the enlargement of the hemisphere the hippocampus is carried backwards and then downwards and forwards on the convexity of the lateral ventricle.

c T— It has connections with the olfactory tracts.

d T— Forming the anterior commissure.

e F— It connects the hippocampal areas.

385 **In the forebrain the:**
  a   falx cerebri lies within the median longitudinal
      fissure.   (   )
  b   tentorium cerebelli lies in the transverse fissure.   (   )
  c   corpus callosum overlies the diencephalon.   (   )

  d   lobes are named after the bones that overlie them.   (   )
  e   cortex has a constant pattern of sulci and gyri.   (   )

386 **On the lateral surface of the cerebral hemisphere:**
  a   the lateral sulcus overlies the insula.   (   )

  b   the central sulcus is continuous over the superior
      border on to the medial surface.   (   )

  c   visual function is primarily represented on the
      lateral aspect of the occipital pole.   (   )

  d   auditory sensation is represented in the inferior
      frontal gyrus.   (   )
  e   speech is subserved by the inferior precentral
      gyrus of the dominant hemisphere.   (   )

387 **In the cerebral isocortex:**
  a   layer I contains an extensive ramification of
      horizontal cells.   (   )
  b   stellate neurons are mainly found in layers III
      and V.   (   )
  c   the external granular layer contains numerous
      small pyramidal cells.   (   )
  d   the very large pyramidal cells of the motor cortex
      are found in layer IV.   (   )
  e   there is a very prominent tangently placed plexus
      in layer IV of the visual cortex.   (   )

a   **T**— Partly separating the two hemispheres.

b   **F**— The occipital lobe of the hemisphere rests on the tentorium
c   **T**   which is attached laterally to the transverse venous
sinuses. The transverse fissure lies between the corpus
callosum dorsally and the diencephalon and midbrain
ventrally.

d   **T**— Namely the frontal, parietal, occipital and temporal lobes.

e   **F**— It is possible usually to define the lateral, central and
calcarine sulci but many of the other surface features are
variable.

a   **T**— The insula is submerged during the enlargement of the
hemisphere.

b   **T**— Motor and somatosensory functions being represented on
the lateral surface are continued on to the medially placed
paracentral lobule.

c   **F**— The cortex overlying the inferior margin and the posterior
half of the superior margin of the calcarine sulcus on the
medial surface of the hemisphere subserve this function.

d   **F**— Auditory sensation is represented in the superior temporal
gyrus.

e   **F**— The inferior frontal gyrus subserves this function.

a   **T**— These cells are small and fusiform; they are prominent in
the newborn.

b   **F**— These neurons are mainly in layers II and IV.

c   **T**— The external and internal granular layers (II and IV) also
contain numerous stellate cells.

d   **F**— These Betz cells are in layer V.

e   **T**— The region is called the striate area.

388 **Fibres of the corpus callosum:**
a unite the olfactory areas of the two sides of the brain.   (   )
b pass in the internal capsule to the frontal lobe.   (   )

c unite adjacent and widely separated gyri in the same hemisphere.   (   )
d unite the two hippocampi.   (   )

e to the occipital lobe form a prominent posterior bundle.   (   )

389 **The internal capsule:**
a lies lateral to the caudate nucleus.   (   )

b carries somatosensory fibres in the posterior limb.   (   )

c carries fibres from the ventroanterior nucleus in the posterior limb.   (   )
d carries pyramidal tract fibres in the posterior limb.   (   )

e carries the visual radiation.   (   )

390 **The caudate nucleus:**
a lies on the convexity of the lateral ventricle.   (   )

b forms part of the corpus striatum.   (   )

c forms a superior relation of the anterior perforated substance.   (   )
d sends most of its efferent fibres in the stria terminalis.   (   )

e has a narrow tail.   (   )

a F— The olfactory (piriform) areas are linked across the midline by the anterior commissure.
b F— The fibres of the corpus callosum are commissural fibres. The internal capsule mostly carries projection fibres.
c F— This is the definition of association fibres.

d F— The hippocampi are joined by the fornix (hippocampal) commissure. The corpus callosum is a commissure joining other cortical areas than those in (a) and (d).
e T— The forceps major.

a T— The thalamus lies medial to the capsule and the lentiform nucleus is lateral.
b T— They pass from the ventroposterior nucleus of the thalamus to the somatosensory postcentral cortex.
c F— These and fibres from the medial nuclei pass to the frontal lobe in the anterior limb of the internal capsule.
d T— They pass from the precentral gyrus to the cranial nerve nuclei and spinal cells. They lie anterior to the sensory fibres in the capsule.
e T— Passing from the lateral geniculate body to the visual cortex.

a F— It lies within the concavity, the head bulging into the lateral wall and floor of the anterior horn of the ventricle.
b T— The name is derived from the grey matter that connects the caudate and lentiform nuclei across the anterior limb of the internal capsule.
c T— The expanded head lies over this area and receives blood vessels through it.
d F— The stria terminalis is the main efferent tract of the amygdala. It runs with the thalamostriate vein in the groove between the thalamus and the caudate nucleus. The caudate nucleus projects fibres to the globus pallidus.
e T— Lying in the roof of the inferior horn of the lateral ventricle.

391   The globus pallidus:
a   forms the lateral part of the lentiform nucleus.   (   )

b   sends efferent fibres to the ventroanterior nucleus
of the thalamus.   (   )
c   lies adjacent to the internal capsule.   (   )

d   receives its main afferent fibres from the claustrum.   (   )

e   is separated from the insula by the claustrum.   (   )

392   The hippocampus:
a   is expanded in the roof of the inferior horn of the
lateral ventricle.   (   )
b   like the septal nuclei, is part of the limbic system.   (   )

c   receives its main afferent fibres through the fornix.   (   )

d   sends efferent fibres to the hypothalamus.   (   )

e   is expanded inferiorly into the amygdaloid body.   (   )

393   The thalamus:
a   is limited anteriorly by the interventricular foramen.   (   )

b   overlies the midbrain anteriorly.   (   )

c   lies in the floor of the body of the lateral ventricle.   (   )

d   forms the medial relation of the anterior limb of
the internal capsule.   (   )
e   is related medially to the third ventricle.

a F— It lies medial to the putamen and they together form the lentiform nucleus.

b T— Also to the ventrolateral nucleus, hypothalamus, subthalamus, substantia nigra and reticular formation.

c T— The anterior and posterior limbs of the internal capsule are medial to the nucleus, the genu being related to the apex of the nucleus.

d F— Afferent fibres come from the caudate nucleus, putamen and substantia nigra. The claustrum is closely linked with the insular cortex.

e F— The claustrum is lateral to the putamen.

a F— It lies on the floor of the inferior horn.

b T— The system also includes the hypothalamus, fornix, cingulate and parahippocampal gyri. It is probably concerned with the emotional and visceral factors of behaviour.

c F— The fornix system is the main efferent pathway of the hippocampus.

d T— Through the fornix mainly and also to the reticular formation.

e F— The amygdaloid body is situated at the end of the tail of the caudate nucleus, over the tip of the inferior horn of the lateral ventricle.

a T— The narrower anterior end of the nucleus has a prominent anterior tubercle on its upper surface near the foramen.

b F— The expanded posterior (pulvinar) region of the thalamus overlies the brainstem. The hypothalamus underlies the thalamus anteriorly.

c T— The caudate nucleus forms the floor of the ventricle laterally and in front.

d F— It lies medial to the posterior limb.

e T— The thalami of the two sides are separated by the narrow cleft of the 3rd ventricle and joined by the interthalamic connection.

394 **In the thalamic nuclei the:**
a anterior nucleus lies within the internal medullary lamina. ( )

b ventroanterior nucleus receives the medial and spinal lemnisci. ( )

c medial geniculate body sends efferent fibres to the superior temporal gyrus. ( )
d anterior nucleus receives the mammillothalamic tract. ( )
e dorsomedial nucleus has extensive reciprocal connections with the frontal cortex. ( )

395 **The hypothalamus:**
a receives afferent fibres from the amygdaloid body through the fornix. ( )

b sends efferent fibres to the anterior lobe of the pituitary in the supra-opticohypophyseal tract. ( )
c sends efferent fibres to the cerebral cortex in the median forebrain bundle. ( )
d is related posteroinferiorly to the posterior perforated substance. ( )

e is linked to the pituitary stalk by the tuberoinfundibular tract. ( )

396 **The pituitary gland (hypophysis cerebri):**
a overlies the posterior ethmoidal air cells. ( )

b sends its venous drainage to the dural sinuses. ( )

c is partly formed as an outgrowth of the primitive foregut. ( )

d posterior lobe secretions affect urine production. ( )

e is an anterior relation of the optic chiasma. ( )

a **T**— The lamina splits the anterior two-thirds of the thalamus, and anterosuperiorly encloses the anterior thalamic nucleus.

b **F**— These fibres pass with the trigeminal lemniscus to the ventroposterior nucleus. The ventroanterior nucleus receives fibres mainly from the globus pallidus.

c **T**— The nucleus relays the auditory impulses which travel in the lateral lemniscus.

d **T**— The efferent fibres pass to the cingulate gyrus.

e **T**— Its links with autonomic and endocrine function serve to integrate visceral and somatic activities.

a **F**— The fibres from the amygdaloid body pass in the stria terminalis. The fornix carries fibres from the hippocampus to the hypothalamus.

b **F**— The tract passes to the posterior lobe.

c **F**— The bundle and the dorsal longitudinal fasciculus pass from the hypothalamus to the midbrain reticular nuclei.

d **F**— This perforated substance is further back in the interpeduncular fossa and underlies the adjacent subthalamus and midbrain.

e **T**— From the tuberal and infundibular nuclei.

a **F**— The body of the sphenoid bone and its air sinus lie inferior to the gland.

b **T**— The cavernous and intercavernous sinuses form a close relation to the gland. A portal circulation also exists between the hypothalamus and the pituitary gland.

c **F**— The anterior and middle lobes are formed from a diverticulum of the stomadeum (Rathke's pouch). The diverticulum is of ectodermal origin, as is the posterior lobe which arises from the forebrain.

d **T**— Also blood pressure, and in the female, they contract the uterine muscle. The anterior lobe secretions affect most other endocrine glands.

e **F**— The stalk is a posterior relation to the optic chiasma.

397   In the epithalamus:
a   the habenular nuclei receive the stria medularis.   (   )

b   lesions of the habenular nuclei can influence metabolic regulation.   (   )

c   the posterior commissure unites the superior colliculi.   (   )

d   the pineal gland has reciprocal innervation with the hypothalamus.   (   )

e   the interpeduncular nuclei receive fibres from a globus pallidus.   (   )

398   The medial relations of the lateral ventricle include the:
a   head of the caudate nucleus.   (   )

b   fornix.   (   )

c   interventricular foramen.   (   )
d   amygdaloid body.   (   )
e   transverse fissure.   (   )

399   The third ventricle:
a   communicates with the 4th ventricle through the interventricular foramen.   (   )

b   is related superiorly to the transverse fissure.   (   )

c   is bounded anteriorly by the lamina terminalis.   (   )

d   is recessed into the mammillary body.   (   )

e   is related inferiorly to the posterior perforated substance.   (   )

a **T**— This narrow bundle passes over the thalamus from the septal nuclei.

b **T**— The nuclei also influence endocrine regulation.

c **T**— Also the posterior thalamic nuclei, the pretectal regions and the medial longitudinal bundles of the two sides.

d **T**— The pineal is a regulator of pituitary activity.

e **F**— These nuclei are part of the subthalamus.

a **F**— This forms the lateral and inferior relation of the anterior horn of the ventricle. The septum pellucidum lies medially.

b **T**— The fibres from the hippocampus lie in the floor of the inferior horn of the ventricle and form the fornix. The medial wall of the ventricle (mainly ependyma) is attached to the fornix and is invaginated as the choroidal fissure.

c **T**— Joining the lateral ventricle to the midline 3rd ventricle.

d **F**— This nucleus lies in front of the apex of the inferior horn.

e **T**— The choroid plexus is invaginated into the ventricle from the tela choroidea in the fissure.

a **F**— The 3rd and 4th ventricles are linked by the cerebral aqueduct. The interventricular foramina link the the 3rd and the lateral ventricles.

b **T**— The fissure lies between the corpus callosum above and the ependymal roof of the diencephalon below. The choroid plexus invaginates the 3rd ventricle from above and each lateral ventricle from the medial side.

c **T**— The anterior commissure is within it and it lies between the corpus callosum above and the optic chiasma below.

d **F**— It is recessed into the optic chiasma and infundibulum in the floor, and within the pineal stalk posterosuperiorly.

e **T**— This lies in the floor behind the mammillary bodies.

400 **In the midbrain the:**
a   inferior brachium carries visual fibres from the
    inferior colliculus to the medial geniculate body.   (   )

b   trochlear nerves have a dorsal decussation around
    the superior colliculus.   (   )

c   cerebral peduncles are separated from the
    tegmentum by a pigmented layer.   (   )
d   superior cerebellar peduncles decussate in the lower
    tegmentum.   (   )

e   superior colliculus communicates with motor
    nuclei of the head and neck.   (   )

401 **In the pons the:**
a   abducent nerve emerges about the middle at the
    junction with the middle cerebellar peduncle.   (   )
b   the facial nerve emerges through the middle
    cerebellar peduncle in the upper pons.   (   )
c   basilar portion is continuous with the cerebral
    peduncles of the midbrain.   (   )

d   nucleus of the tractus solitarius lies lateral to the
    facial motor nucleus.   (   )

e   fibres from the dorsal and ventral cochlear nuclei
    lie in the lower pons and form the trapezoid body.   (   )

402 **In the pons the:**
a   vestibulospinal tract arises from the larger medial
    part of the vestibular nuclei.   (   )

b   trapezoid body sends its fibres into the medial
    lemniscus.   (   )
c   medial longitudinal fasciculus lies dorsally near
    the midline in the floor of the 4th ventricle.   (   )

d   medial lemniscus becomes more laterally and
    ventrally placed as it ascends.   (   )
e   vagus nerve emerges below the abducent.   (   )

a **F**— The inferior brachium carries auditory fibres between these centres. Visual fibres pass in the less well defined ridge from the superior colliculus to the lateral geniculate body.

b **F**— The dorsal decussation lies below the inferior colliculi. The oculomotor nerves leave ventrally at the level of the superior colliculi.

c **T**— The substantia nigra. The region dorsal to the aqueduct is known as the tectum.

d **T**— Passing to the red nucleus and the thalamus. The red nucleus receives fibres from the globus pallidus and sends efferent fibres to the reticular formation of the brain stem, and to the thalamus.

e **T**— Through the medial longitudinal bundle.

a **F**— This is the site of exit of the trigeminal nerve. The abducent, facial and vestibulocochlear nerves (medial to

b **F** lateral) emerge at the lower border of the pons.

c **T**— The descending pyramidal fibres are split up by the transversely running fibres passing to the middle cerebellar peduncle.

d **T**— The facial motor fibres make a dorsal loop over the abducent nucleus before emerging. Joining the facial nerve are taste fibres (to the nucleus of the tractus solitarius) and the parasympathetic fibres from the upper part of the salivary nucleus.

e **T**— These fibres arise in the cochlear nuclei on the floor of the lateral recess of the 4th ventricle. Many pass up to the medial geniculate body in the lateral lemniscus.

a **F**— The tract arises from the larger lateral part of the nuclei and ends amongst the anterior horn cells of the same side mainly in the spinal cord.

b **F**— The fibres pass in the lateral lemniscus to the medial geniculate body and the inferior colliculus.

c **T**— The two bundles communicate through the posterior commissure. They receive fibres from the vestibular nuclei, and send fibres to the nuclei supplying the ocular muscles, and the motor nuclei of the cervical spinal cord.

d **T**— The spinal lemniscus lies on its lateral side, and the lateral lemniscus is lateral to the whole tract.

e **F**— The vagus nerve emerges in the medulla.

403   The medulla has:
a   an anterior median fissure running uninterruptedly throughout its length.   ( )
b   the hypoglossal nerve rootlets emerging between the pyramid and the olive.   ( )
c   the inferior medullary velum as a dorsal relation.   ( )
d   the dorsally placed gracile nucleus lying lateral to the cuneate nucleus.   ( )
e   the spinal nucleus of the trigeminal nerve situated posterolaterally.   ( )

404   In the medulla the:
a   olivary efferent fibres decussate as internal arcuate fibres.   ( )
b   dorsal vagal nucleus lies medial to the hypoglossal nucleus.   ( )
c   nucleus ambiguus lies deeply between the hypoglossal and dorsal vagal nuclei.   ( )
d   anterior spinocerebellar tract ascends into the midbrain and enters the superior cerebellar peduncle of the same side.   ( )
e   posterior spinocerebellar tract passes uncrossed in the inferior cerebellar peduncle.   ( )

405   In the cerebellum the:
a   primary fissure divides the flocculonodular lobe from the middle lobe.   ( )
b   Purkinje cells are situated in the middle of the three cortical layers.   ( )
c   Purkinje fibres of the vermis project on to the dentate nucleus.   ( )
d   Purkinje fibres of the paravermal zone project on to the nucleus interpositum.   ( )
e   horizontal fissure divides the anterior and middle lobes.   ( )

a F— The fissure is crossed by the decussation of the pyramids in the lower part.

b T— The vagus and glossopharyngeal rootlets emerge dorsal to the olive, between it and the inferior cerebellar peduncle.

c T— The roof of the open medulla is completed above by the cerebellum and the superior medullary velum.

d F— The gracile nucleus relays impulses from the lower limb and is medial to the cuneate which is concerned with the upper limb. They form prominent elevations in the lower medulla, their fibres decussate as the internal arcuate fibres and form the medial lemniscus.

e T— It extends throughout the length of the medulla.

a T— They pass into the inferior cerebellar peduncle. Other internal arcuate fibres are the main somatosensory decussation forming the medial lemniscus.

b F— The hypoglossal nucleus lies near the midline in the floor of the 4th ventricle and the vagal nucleus is just lateral to it.

c T— Fibres from the nucleus ambiguus pass in the vagus and glossopharyngeal nerves and mainly supply muscles derived from the 4th and 6th pharyngeal arch mesenchyme.

d T— It passes mainly to the vermis and anterior lobe of the cerebellum.

e T

a F— The primary fissure divides the anterior and middle lobes. The posterolateral fissure separates the flocculonodular lobe.

b T— It has inner granular and outer molecular layers. Only about one-sixth of the markedly uniform convoluted surface is visible externally.

c F— The vermis projects to the fastigial nucleus. The large lateral part of the hemisphere projects to the dentate nucleus.

d T— This nucleus is made up of the globose and emboliform nuclei.

e F— The fissure divides the posterior lobe into approximately equal inferior and superior halves.

406   Cerebellar afferent fibres from the:
a   cerebral cortex pass mainly to the flocculonodular
    lobe of the opposite side.   (   )
b   vestibular nuclei pass mainly to the anterior lobe.   (   )

c   olivary nuclei pass to all parts of the cerebellum.   (   )

d   posterior spinocerebellar tract pass to the vermis
    and paravermal zone of the anterior and middle
    lobes.   (   )
e   dorsal column of the upper spinal cord pass to the
    vermis and paravermal zone of the anterior and
    middle lobes.   (   )

407   Cerebellar efferent fibres:
a   from the dentate nucleus pass to the ventrolateral
    nucleus of the thalamus of the opposite side.   (   )

b   from the emboliform nucleus pass to the globus
    pallidus on the opposite side.   (   )

c   from the fastigial nucleus pass to the vestibular
    nuclei.   (   )

d   are responsible for initiating voluntary movement.   (   )

e   within the middle cerebellar peduncle pass to the
    vestibular nuclei.   (   )

408   The 4th ventricle:
a   is limited superiorly by the superior cerebellar
    peduncles.   (   )
b   choroid plexus is formed by invagination of the
    superior medullary velum.   (   )
c   is recessed laterally around the superior cerebellar
    peduncles.   (   )
d   has the facial colliculus near the midline rostral
    to the striae medullares.   (   )

e   is bounded inferiorly by the pyramids.   (   )

a **F**— They synapse in the pontine nuclei and cross to all parts of the cerebellum other than the flocculonodular lobe. The
b **F** flocculonodular lobe receives fibres from the vestibular nuclei.
c **T**— Decussating as the upper group of internal arcuate fibres and passing through the inferior cerebellar peduncle.
d **T**— The fibres originate in the cells of the thoracic nucleus and pass uncrossed in the inferior cerebellar peduncle.

e **T**— They synapse in the accessory cuneate nucleus and pass uncrossed in the inferior cerebellar peduncle.

a **T**— The impulses are relayed to the cerebral cortex. Other impulses are relayed in the red nucleus and descend into the cord.
b **T**— Fibres from the dentate nucleus and nucleus interpositum pass through the superior cerebellar peduncle and decussate in the lower midbrain. They end in the red nucleus, ventrolateral thalamic nucleus and globus pallidus.
c **T**— Fibres pass through the superior and inferior cerebellar peduncles. Some also end in the reticular nuclei of the pons and the medulla.
d **F**— The cerebellum influences the pattern of a movement which has been initiated by the cerebrum. The effects of cerebellar disease are seen on the same side as the lesion.
e **F**— This peduncle carries predominantly pontocerebellar fibres.

a **T**— The superior medullary velum, passing between the peduncles, forms the upper roof of the ventricle.
b **F**— The invagination is of the inferior medullary velum.

c **F**— The lateral recess is around the inferior cerebellar peduncles. Each has an opening at its tip.
d **T**— The ventricle has the hypoglossal and vagal triangles and the vestibular areas overlying their respective nuclei, caudal to the striae.
e **F**— The inferior boundary is the gracile and cuneate tubercles.

409   In the spinal cord the:
a   grey matter of the thoracic segment is
proportionately larger than the cervical.   (   )

b   gelatinous substances overly the posterior horn
of grey matter.   (   )
c   filum terminale is formed at the lower border of
the 4th lumbar vertebra.   (   )

d   lateral horn gives rise to preganglionic autonomic
nerve fibres.   (   )
e   nucleus proprius makes up most of the dorsal horn.   (   )

410   The dorsal root ganglion contains the cell bodies of the:
a   dorsal column of the spinal cord.   (   )
b   anterior spinocerebellar tract.   (   )

c   dorsolateral tract.   (   )

d   lateral spinothalamic tract.   (   )

e   reticulospinal tract.   (-)

411   The spinal afferent:
a   touch fibres have their cell bodies (primary neurons)
in the dorsal root ganglia.   (   )
b   pressure fibres have their cell bodies in the dorsal
root ganglion.   (   )

c   temperature fibres comprise a thinly myelinated
lateral division of the dorsal root.   (   )
d   pain fibres pass to the ventroposterior nucleus of
the thalamus.   (   )

e   proprioceptive fibres are partly carried in the dorsal
column.   (   )

a **F**— The grey matter of the cervical and lumbar cord is increased. The enlargements correspond to the large nerve roots supplying the limbs.

b **T**— It is a region of small cells.

c **F**— The spinal cord ends at the upper border of the second lumbar vertebra in the adult. The dural sac ends at the level of the second piece of the sacrum and the vertebral canal ends at the sacral hiatus.

d **T**— It is found in the thoracic and sacral regions.

e **T**— It contains cell bodies of secondary neurons subserving touch, pain and temperature.

a **T**— The fibres ascend to the gracile and cuneate nuclei.

b **F**— The cell bodies of this tract lie in the posterior horn of the opposite side. The fibres pass to the cerebellum in the superior cerebellar peduncle.

c **T**— Some fibres in the dorsolateral tract arise in the dorsal root ganglion but most arise from neurons in the adjacent grey matter.

d **F**— The cell bodies of the tract lie in the posterior horn of the opposite side. The fibres cross in the anterior white commissure and pass to the thalamus in the spinal lemniscus.

e **F**— This contains extrapyramidal motor fibres.

a **T**— These fibres pass in the dorsal column and end in the gracile and cuneate nuclei. Fibres from these secondary neurons cross the midline and form the medial lemniscus, passing to the ventroposterior nucleus of the thalamus. A third set of fibres pass to the postcentral gyrus.

b **T**

c **T**— The medial division is heavily myelinated and conveys touch pain, vibration and proprioception.

d **T**— Many pain impulses are relayed in the posterior horn grey matter and then travel to the thalamus in the spinothalamic tracts of the opposite side of the cord. Impulses are relayed to the postcentral cortical gyrus. A further series of fibres have a diffuse representation through the reticular formation.

e **T**— These fibres mainly synapse in the accessory cuneate nucleus. Fibres from this nucleus pass uncrossed in the inferior cerebellar peduncle and take part in reflex control of movement. Some proprioceptive information reaches consciousness along with touch and pressure information.

412 **In the efferent pathways of the central nervous system the:**

a tectospinal pathways facilitate control of balance. ( )

b corticospinal tract contains approximately 100 000 fibres. ( )

c corticospinal fibres usually end directly on the anterior horn cells. ( )

d corticospinal fibres are predominantly crossed. ( )

e reticulospinal tract receives additional fibres from the cerebellum and red nucleus. ( )

413 **In the cranial nerve nuclei the:**

a general somatic efferent column innervates the muscles of the larynx. (

b special visceral efferent column innervates muscles derived from pharyngeal arch mesoderm. (

c parasympathetic fibres originate in the trigeminal nerve nucleus. (

d special visceral afferent column carries sensory fibres from the proximal pharynx. (

e general somatic afferent column carries sensory fibres in the facial nerve. (

414 **In the cranial dura mater the:**

a outer layer is infolded to form the falx cerebri. (

b tentorium cerebelli is formed from the endocranial layer. (

c free edge of the tentorium cerebelli passes forwards to the anterior clinoid process. (

d innervation is partly from the vagus nerve. (

e cranial nerves receive a sheath from the cerebral layer as they leave the skull. (

a F— They facilitate visual and auditory motor reflexes. Balance is controlled through the vestibulospinal pathways.

b F— There are approximately 1 million fibres, 60% arising from the precentral cortex.

c F— A few fibres end in this way, these being mostly to muscles performing precise movements, such as in the hand. The majority of fibres synapse through an interneuron.

d T— However, motor neurons of the upper face, tongue, pharynx and larynx receive ipsi and contralateral innervation through corticobulbar fibres.

e T— These fibres mainly innervate axial and proximal limb musculature, and are concerned with the control of muscle tone, posture and programmed limb movements, such as those used for locomotion.

a T— This column comprises the oculogyric and hypoglossal nerves.

b T— These fibres are carried in the trigeminal, facial, glossopharyngeal, vagus and accessory nerves.

c F— General visceral, afferent and efferent fibres are carried in the oculomotor, facial, glossopharyngeal and vagus nerves.

d F— This column carries taste fibres in the facial, glossopharyngeal and vagus nerves.

e F— These fibres, derived from face, scalp, nose, nasal sinuses, mouth and teeth, are carried in the trigeminal nerve.

a F— The outer (endocranial) layer is the periosteum of the bone
b F and does not leave it. It is continuous with the outer periosteum through the sutures. The dural folds are formed from the inner (cerebral) layer.

c T— The attached border passes along the apex of the petrous temporal bone to the posterior clinoid process.

d T— Also from the trigeminal, glossopharyngeal and upper three cervical nerves.

e T— That formed around the optic nerve reaches the back of the eyeball.

415 The spinal dura mater:
a   is continuous with the inner layer of the cranial
    dura mater.   (   )
b   has a double layer for most of its course.   (   )
c   extends downwards to the level of the 2nd
    sacral vertebra.   (   )

d   is pierced separately by the dorsal and ventral
    roots of the spinal nerves.   (   )
e   is partly stabilised within the vertebral canal by the
    dentate ligaments.   (   )

416 The pia mater:
a   extends into the posterior median sulcus of the
    spinal cord.   (   )

b   is invaginated into the cerebral ventricles.   (   )

c   has an opening over the inferior horn of each
    lateral ventricle.   (   )

d   extends forwards as a fold beneath the corpus
    callosum.   (   )

e   extends with the dural sac to the level of the
    2nd sacral vertebra.   (   )

417 In the circulation of the cerebrospinal fluid:
a   production is mainly by active secretion.   (   )

b   reabsorption is partly through spinal perineural
    lymph vessels and veins.   (   )

c   blockage within the ventricular system produces
    communicating hydrocephalus.   (   )

d   the arachnoid granulations pierce the inner layer
    of dura mater.   (   )
e   the ventricular system communicates with the
    subarachnoid space in the tela choroidea.   (   )

a T— The dura is separated from the bony-ligamentous vertebral canal by the fat-filled epidural space.

b F— There is a single layer throughout.

c T— The spinal cord ends opposite the second lumbar vertebra and the lower dural sheath contains the cauda equina and lumbar cistern. The filum terminale ends on the back of the coccyx.

d T— The dura ensheaths these and the spinal nerve as far as the intervertebral foramen.

e F— The ligaments are pial structures stabilising the spinal cord within the dural sac. The dural sheath is stabilised by the emerging nerves and the filum terminale.

a F— The pia mater extends into the anterior median fissure and the cerebral sulci. It also ensheaths the origins of the spinal and cranial nerves.

b T— The pia mater and the adjacent thin ependymal layer form the choroid plexus of each ventricle.

c F— A medial and two lateral apertures in the roof of the 4th ventricle allow cerebrospinal fluid to pass from the ventricular system into the subarachnoid space.

d T— This fold into the transverse fissure is known as the tela choroidea. Lateral and inferior extensions from it pass into the lateral and 3rd ventricles and form the choroid plexuses of these ventricles.

e F— The pia mater ends with the spinal cord, opposite the 2nd lumbar vertebra.

a T— The modified ependymal cells of the choroid plexus are involved in this process.

b T— But the main absorption is through the arachnoid granulations in the superior sagittal sinus and its lateral recesses.

c F— Blockage at this level causes dilatation of the ventricular system which is known as internal hydrocephalus. The communicating form is due to blockage of the arachnoid granulations.

d T— These then come into contact with the endothelium of the venous sinuses.

e F— The communications are in the roof of the 4th ventricle.

418 **The internal carotid artery:**

a enters the cranium through the squamous
temporal bone. ( )

b lies within the dural coverings of the cavernous
sinus. ( )

c gives a branch to the choroid plexus of the 3rd
ventricle. ( )

d pierces the diaphragma sella medial to the optic
nerve. ( )

e has an ophthalmic branch entering the orbit through
the superior orbital fissure. ( )

419 **The vertebral artery:**

a enters the cranial cavity through the posterior
condylar canal. ( )

b unites with its fellow of the opposite side at the
upper border of the pons to form the basilar artery. ( )

c sends branches to the spinal cord from within the
cranial cavity. ( )

d supplies the choroidal plexus of the 4th ventricle. ( )

e supplies the cerebellar vermis through its superior
cerebellar branch. ( )

420 **The basilar artery:**

a divides distally into two superior cerebellar arteries. ( )

b gives branches to the lateral and 3rd ventricles. ( )

c supplies both the motor and somatosensory cortical
areas. ( )

d supplies the auditory area of cortex. ( )

e supplies branches to the inner ear. ( )

a **F**— The carotid canal lies within the petrous temporal bone.

b **T**— In company with the abducent and other nerves, and covered by the venous endothelium.

c **F**— Its anterior choroidal branch supplies the inferior horn of the lateral ventricle.

d **F**— The artery lies lateral to the optic nerve.

e **F**— Its ophthalmic branch passes into the optic canal within the dural sheath of the optic nerve.

a **F**— The artery passes through the foramen magnum.

b **F**— The basilar artery is formed at the lower border of the pons.

c **T**— The anterior spinal artery comes directly from the vertebral artery and the posterior spinal artery from its posterior inferior cerebellar branch.

d **T**— The choroidal artery comes from the posterior inferior cerebellar artery.

e **F**— This is a branch of the basilar artery.

a **F**— Its terminal branches are the two posterior cerebral arteries.

b **T**— The posterior choroidal branch of the posterior cerebral artery enters the tela choroidea and supplies these ventricles.

c **F**— Most of the pre- and postcentral gyri and the superior temporal gyrus are supplied by the middle cerebral artery.

d **F**— The posterior cerebral artery supplies the occipital pole with its visual areas.

e **T**— The labyrinthine artery passes through the internal acoustic meatus.

421 **In the cerebral venous drainage the:**
  a   superior cerebral veins pass to the inferior sagittal sinus. ( )

  b   anterior cerebral vein joins the deep middle cerebral vein. ( )
  c   choroidal veins from the lateral and 3rd ventricles pass into the cavernous sinuses. ( )
  d   great cerebral vein is formed from the internal cerebral vein of each side. ( )
  e   great cerebral vein opens into the cavernous sinus. ( )

422 **In the cranial venous sinuses the:**
  a   superior sagittal sinus passes backwards to the internal occipital protuberance. ( )
  b   inferior sagittal sinus passes backwards to the free edge of the tentorium cerebelli. ( )
  c   sigmoid sinus grooves the inner surface of the mastoid process. ( )
  d   inferior petrosal sinus grooves the parieto-occipital suture. ( )
  e   straight sinus runs posteriorly within the tentorium cerebelli. ( )

423 **The cavernous sinus is related:**
  a   superiorly to the pituitary gland. ( )
  b   laterally to the thalamus. ( )

  c   posteriorly to the facial nerve. ( )

  d   anteriorly to the superior orbital fissure. ( )

  e   inferiorly to the ethmoidal air sinus. ( )

a F— The veins pass to the superior sagittal sinus. They can be easily damaged by anteroposterior deceleration injuries of the head.

b T— They form the basal vein which passes over the midbrain to join the great cerebral vein.

c F— They join the internal cerebral vein which also receives the thalamostriate vein.

d T— It lies in the tela choroidea in the transverse fissure.

e F— It opens into the straight sinus.

a T— It usually joins the right transverse sinus.

b T— Where it joins the straight sinus.

c T— This relation is important in the spread of infection and in surgery of this region.

d F— It grooves the temporo-occipital suture and unites the cavernous sinus to the internal jugular vein.

e T— It usually joins the left transverse sinus.

a F— It is a lateral relation of the gland.

b F— Its lateral relation is the medial surface of the temporal lobe.

c F— The facial nerve lies in the posterior cranial fossa. The abducent nerve enters the sinus posteriorly.

d T— The ophthalmic veins and the oculomotor and trochlear nerves, and branches of the ophthalmic division of the trigeminal nerve are closely related to the sinus in this region.

e F— It lies on the body of the sphenoid bone.

5407847113923918

12/2022

420

03335718316